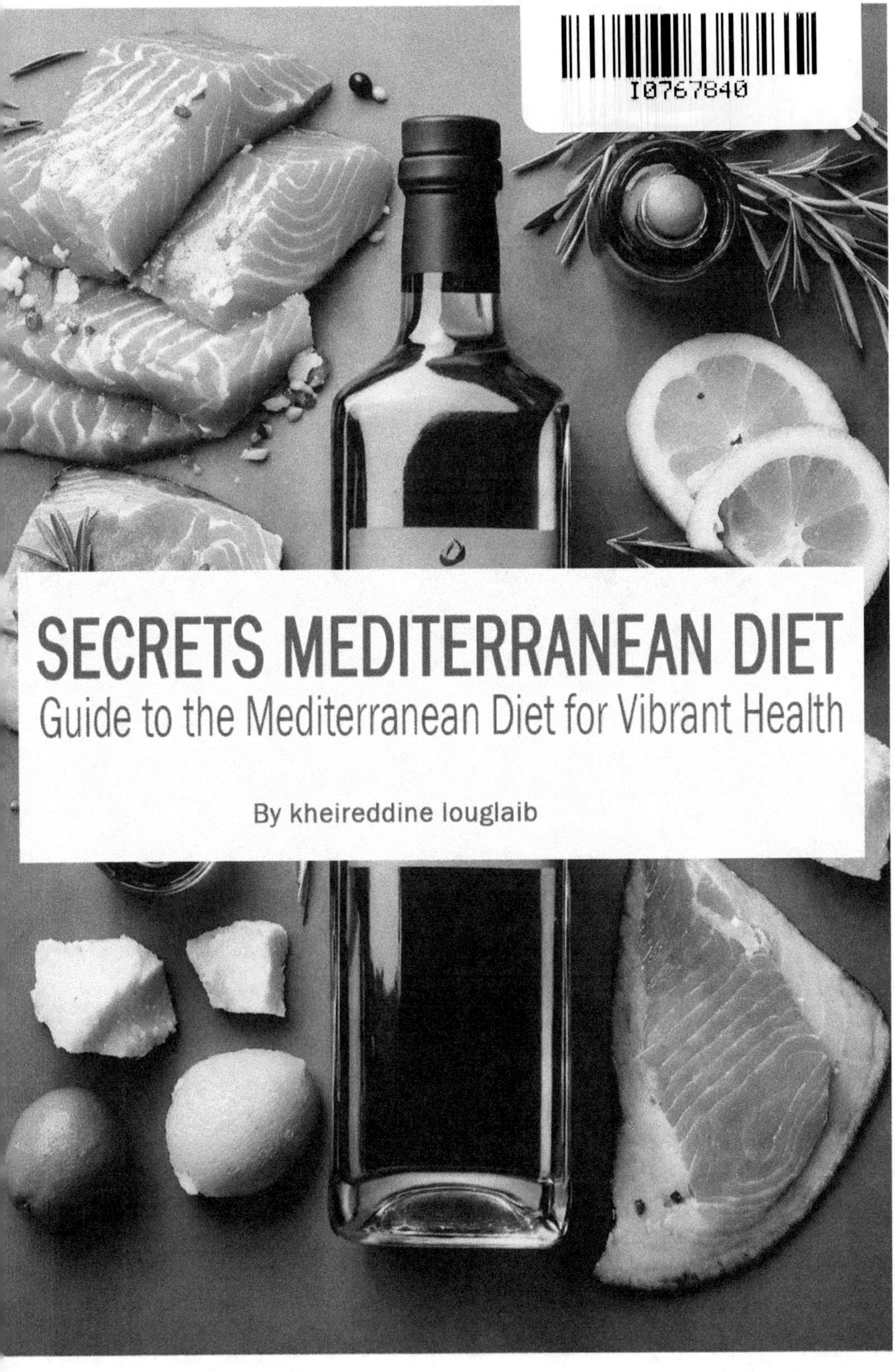

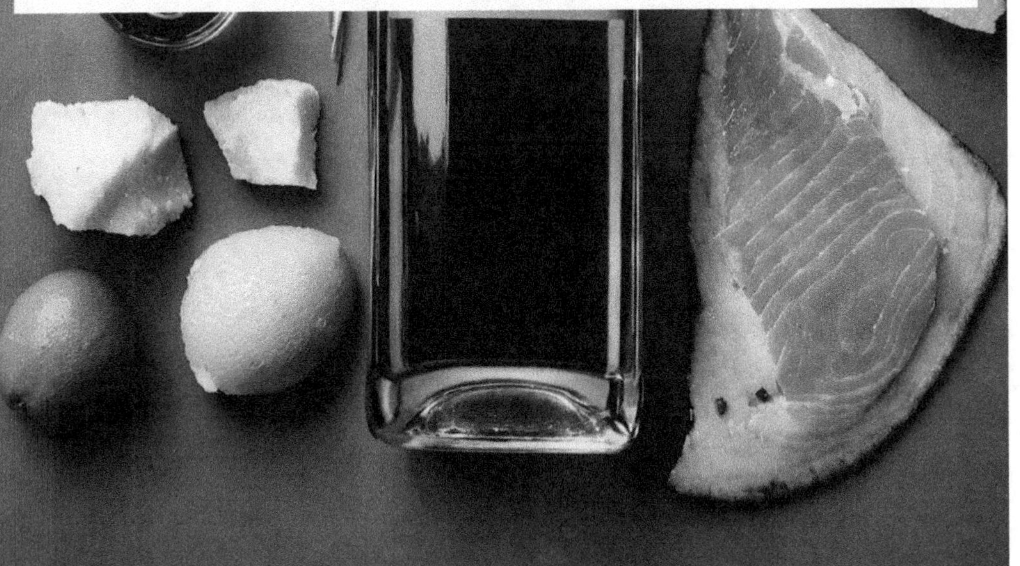

SECRETS MEDITERRANEAN DIET

Guide to the Mediterranean Diet for Vibrant Health

By kheireddine louglaib

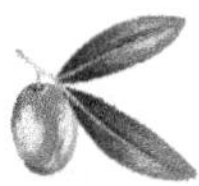

*** Contents ***

Chapter 1: Understanding the Mediterranean Diet

In this chapter, we will discuss the principles of the Mediterranean diet and how it promotes health and well-being. We will explore the history and culture behind this diet and the key components of a Mediterranean diet meal plan.

Chapter 2: Kitchen Essentials for Mediterranean Cooking

This chapter will provide an overview of the essential tools and ingredients needed for cooking Mediterranean cuisine. We will discuss the importance of quality ingredients, including olive oil, herbs, and spices, and provide tips for selecting and storing fresh produce.

Chapter 3: Appetizers and Snacks

In this chapter, we will explore a variety of flavorful and healthy appetizers and snacks that are perfect for entertaining or as a quick bite. Recipes will include hummus, tzatziki, stuffed grape leaves, and more.

Chapter 4: Soups and Salads

This chapter will feature hearty and nutritious soups and salads that are a staple of the Mediterranean diet. Recipes will include lentil soup, Greek salad, and Panzanella.

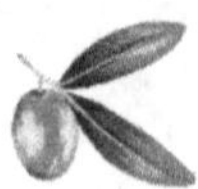

Chapter 5: Main Dishes

The main dishes chapter will showcase a variety of delicious and healthy Mediterranean meals, including seafood, poultry, and vegetarian options. Recipes will include grilled fish, chicken souvlaki, and vegetable lasagna.

Chapter 6: Sides and Accompaniments

This chapter will provide recipes for healthy and flavorful Mediterranean side dishes, such as roasted vegetables, couscous, and quinoa.

Chapter 7: Desserts and Sweets

In this chapter, we will explore sweet treats that are inspired by the Mediterranean diet. Recipes will include baklava, fruit sorbet, and almond cookies.

Chapter 8: Meal Planning and Prep

This chapter will provide tips and strategies for meal planning and prepping, including batch cooking and freezer-friendly recipes. We will also discuss how to make the most of leftovers and reduce food waste.

Conclusion:

The Mediterranean diet is more than just a way of eating, it's a lifestyle. This cookbook is a comprehensive guide to cooking delicious and healthy Mediterranean meals at home. With a focus on whole, nutrient-dense foods, this diet can help you feel your best and reduce your risk of chronic disease. Let this cookbook be your guide to a healthier and more flavorful way of eating.

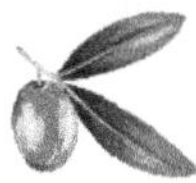

*** Introduction ***

The Mediterranean diet has been gaining popularity in recent years due to its numerous health benefits. This diet is based on the traditional foods and cooking styles of the Mediterranean region, which includes countries like Greece, Italy, Spain, and Turkey. The Mediterranean diet emphasizes whole, nutrient-dense foods like fruits, vegetables, whole grains, and healthy fats. It has been linked to reduced risk of chronic diseases like heart disease, diabetes, and certain types of cancer. This cookbook is a comprehensive guide to cooking delicious and healthy Mediterranean meals at home.

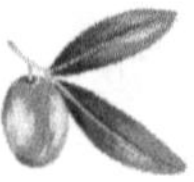

Chapter 1

Understanding the Mediterranean Diet

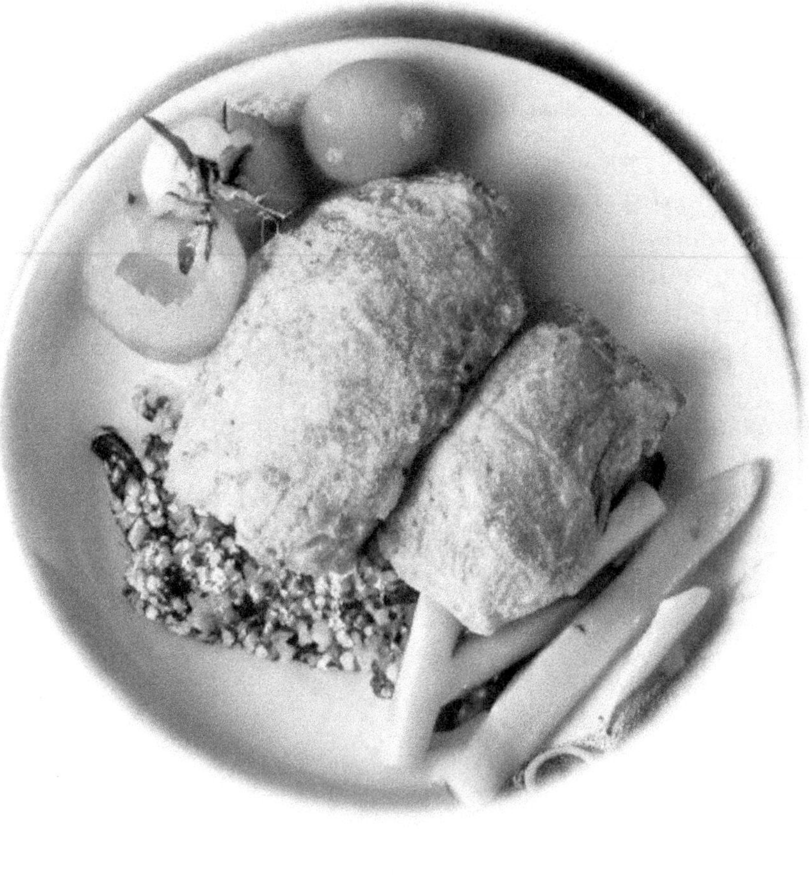

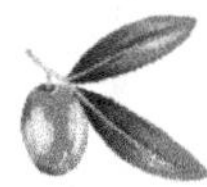

The Mediterranean diet is based on the traditional foods and cooking styles of the Mediterranean region, which emphasizes whole, nutrient-dense foods like fruits, vegetables, whole grains, legumes, nuts, and healthy fats. The key principles of the Mediterranean diet include:

Plant-based foods: The Mediterranean diet emphasizes a variety of plant-based foods, including fruits, vegetables, whole grains, legumes, nuts, and seeds. These foods are rich in fiber, vitamins, minerals, and antioxidants, which can help reduce inflammation and prevent chronic diseases.

Healthy fats: The Mediterranean diet is high in healthy fats like olive oil, nuts, and fatty fish. These fats are rich in omega-3 fatty acids, which have been linked to reduced risk of heart disease and other chronic diseases

Lean protein: The Mediterranean diet includes lean protein sources like fish, poultry, and legumes, which are lower in saturated fat than red meat.

Limited red meat: Red meat is consumed in moderation in the Mediterranean diet, and is often replaced with plant-based protein sources.

Herbs and spices: The Mediterranean diet uses herbs and spices to add flavor to meals, rather than relying on salt and processed condiments.

Moderate alcohol intake: The Mediterranean diet includes moderate alcohol consumption, usually in the form of red wine.

Research has shown that following the Mediterranean diet can lead to numerous health benefits, including reduced risk of heart disease, stroke, diabetes, and certain types of

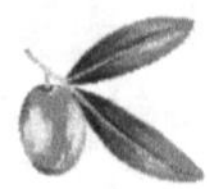

cancer. It can also improve cognitive function, reduce inflammation, and promote longevity.

Here are some additional details on the health benefits of the Mediterranean diet:

Reduced risk of heart disease: The Mediterranean diet has been shown to reduce the risk of heart disease by lowering levels of LDL **("bad")** cholesterol, reducing blood pressure, and improving overall heart health.

Improved brain function: The Mediterranean diet has been linked to better cognitive function and a reduced risk of neurodegenerative diseases like Alzheimer's and Parkinson's.

Better weight management: The Mediterranean diet emphasizes whole, nutrient-dense foods that are low in calories but high in fiber and protein, which can help with weight management.

Reduced inflammation: The Mediterranean diet is rich in anti-inflammatory foods like fruits, vegetables, nuts, and fatty fish, which can help reduce inflammation in the body.

Lower risk of certain types of cancer: Studies have shown that the Mediterranean diet may reduce the risk of certain types of cancer, including breast and colon cancer.

Improved gut health: The Mediterranean diet is high in fiber and prebiotic foods like onions, garlic, and artichokes, which can promote a healthy gut microbiome.

Overall, the Mediterranean diet is a healthy and sustainable way of eating that emphasizes whole, nutrient-dense foods and has been linked to numerous health benefits.

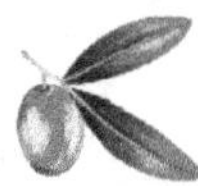

What are some examples of Mediterranean diet meals?

Here are some examples of Mediterranean diet meals:

***** Breakfast *****

- Greek yogurt topped with fresh berries, nuts, and honey

- Omelette with spinach, tomatoes, and feta cheese

- Whole-grain toast with avocado, smoked salmon, and a poached egg

***** Lunch *****

- Mediterranean salad with mixed greens, cherry tomatoes, olives, cucumbers, feta cheese, and a lemon-herb vinaigrette

- Grilled chicken or fish with roasted vegetables and quinoa or brown rice

- Chickpea and vegetable soup with a side of whole-grain bread

***** Dinner *****

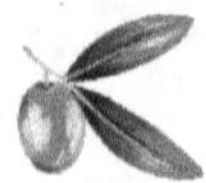

- Grilled shrimp or chicken kebabs with a Greek salad and tzatziki sauce

- Baked salmon with roasted sweet potatoes and Brussels sprouts

- Vegetable lasagna with a side of garlic bread and a mixed green salad.

***** Snacks *****

- Hummus with carrot sticks or whole-grain pita chips

- Apple slices with almond butter

- Roasted chickpeas seasoned with herbs and spices.

***** Dessert *****

- Fresh fruit salad with mint and a drizzle of honey

- Frozen yogurt topped with chopped nuts and fresh berries

- Greek yogurt with honey and walnuts

These are just a few examples of Mediterranean diet meals, but the options are endless. The key is to focus on whole, nutrient-dense foods and to use herbs, spices, and healthy fats to add flavor to meals.

Here are some easy Mediterranean diet recipes that you can prepare at home:

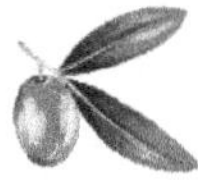

****** <u>Greek Salad</u> ******

Ingredients:

- 2 cups mixed greens
- 1/2 cup cherry tomatoes, halved
- 1/4 cup sliced red onion
- 1/4 cup crumbled feta cheese
- 1/4 cup Kalamata olives
- 2 tbsp extra-virgin olive oil
- 1 tbsp red wine vinegar
- Salt and pepper to taste

*** Instructions:

01- Combine the mixed greens, cherry tomatoes, red onion, feta cheese, and Kalamata olives in a bowl.

02- In a separate bowl, whisk together the olive oil, red wine vinegar, salt, and pepper.

03- Drizzle the dressing over the salad and toss to combine.

****** <u>Baked Salmon with Lemon and Herbs</u> *****

Ingredients:

- 4 salmon fillets
- 2 tbsp extra-virgin olive oil
- 2 tbsp fresh lemon juice
- 2 cloves garlic, minced
- 1 tsp dried oregano

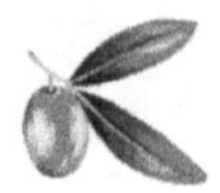

- Salt and pepper to taste

Instructions:

01- Preheat the oven to 400°F (200°C).

02- In a small bowl, whisk together the olive oil, lemon juice, garlic, oregano, salt, and pepper.

03- Place the salmon fillets in a baking dish and pour the marinade over them.

04- Bake for 10-12 minutes, or until the salmon is cooked through.

**** <u>Chickpea and Vegetable Stew</u> ***

Ingredients:

- 1 tbsp extra-virgin olive oil
- 1 yellow onion, diced
- 2 cloves garlic, minced
- 1 red bell pepper, diced
- 1 zucchini, diced
- 1 cup diced tomatoes
- 1 can chickpeas, drained and rinsed
- 2 cups vegetable broth
- 1 tsp dried oregano
- Salt and pepper to taste

Instructions:

01- Heat the olive oil in a large pot over medium heat.

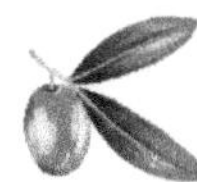

02- Add the onion and garlic and sauté for 2-3 minutes, or until the onion is translucent.

03- Add the red bell pepper and zucchini and sauté for another 5 minutes.

04- Add the diced tomatoes, chickpeas, vegetable broth, oregano, salt, and pepper, and bring to a boil.

05- Reduce the heat and simmer for 10-15 minutes, or until the vegetables are tender.

These easy Mediterranean diet recipes are all packed with flavor and nutrients and can be enjoyed for any meal of the day.

Mediterranean diet recipes that are vegetarian?

Here are some additional vegetarian Mediterranean diet recipes:

*** <u>Mediterranean Quinoa Salad</u> ***

Ingredients:

- 2 cups cooked quinoa
- 1 can chickpeas, drained and rinsed
- 1 cucumber, diced
- 1 red bell pepper, diced
- 1/2 red onion, diced
- 1/4 cup chopped fresh parsley
- 1/4 cup chopped fresh mint

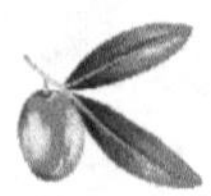

- 1/4 cup extra-virgin olive oil
- 2 tbsp red wine vinegar
- Salt and pepper to taste

Instructions:

01- In a large bowl, combine the cooked quinoa, chickpeas, cucumber, red bell pepper, red onion, parsley, and mint.

03- In a small bowl, whisk together the olive oil, red wine vinegar, salt, and pepper.

04- Drizzle the dressing over the salad and toss to combine.

*** <u>Roasted Vegetable and Feta Tart</u> ***

Ingredients:

- 1 sheet frozen puff pastry, thawed
- 1 small zucchini, sliced
- 1 small yellow squash, sliced
- 1 red bell pepper, sliced
- 1 red onion, sliced
- 1/2 cup crumbled feta cheese
- 2 tbsp extra-virgin olive oil
- Salt and pepper to taste

Instructions:

01- Preheat the oven to 400°F (200°C).

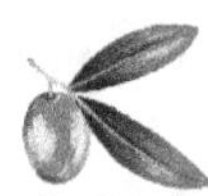

02- Roll out the puff pastry on a lightly floured surface and transfer to a baking sheet.

03- In a large bowl, toss the sliced vegetables with olive oil, salt, and pepper.

04- Arrange the vegetables on top of the puff pastry, leaving a 1-inch border around the edges.

05- Sprinkle the feta cheese over the vegetables.

06-Bake for 20-25 minutes, or until the puff pastry is golden brown and the vegetables are tender.

*** <u>**Mediterranean Veggie Wraps**</u> ***

Ingredients:

- 4 whole-wheat tortillas
- 1/2 cup hummus
- 1/2 cup chopped cucumber
- 1/2 cup chopped cherry tomatoes
- 1/4 cup chopped red onion
- 1/4 cup crumbled feta cheese
- 2 tbsp chopped fresh parsley
- Salt and pepper to taste

Instructions:

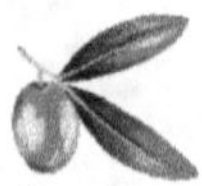

01- Lay out the tortillas and spread a generous amount of hummus on each one.

02-Divide the chopped cucumber, cherry tomatoes, red onion, feta cheese, and parsley among the tortillas.

03- Season with salt and pepper to taste.

04- Roll up the tortillas and slice them in half.

   These vegetarian Mediterranean diet recipes are easy to prepare and packed with flavor and nutrients. Enjoy!

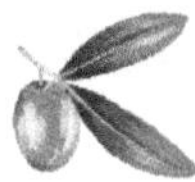

Chapter 2

Kitchen Essentials for Mediterranean Cooking

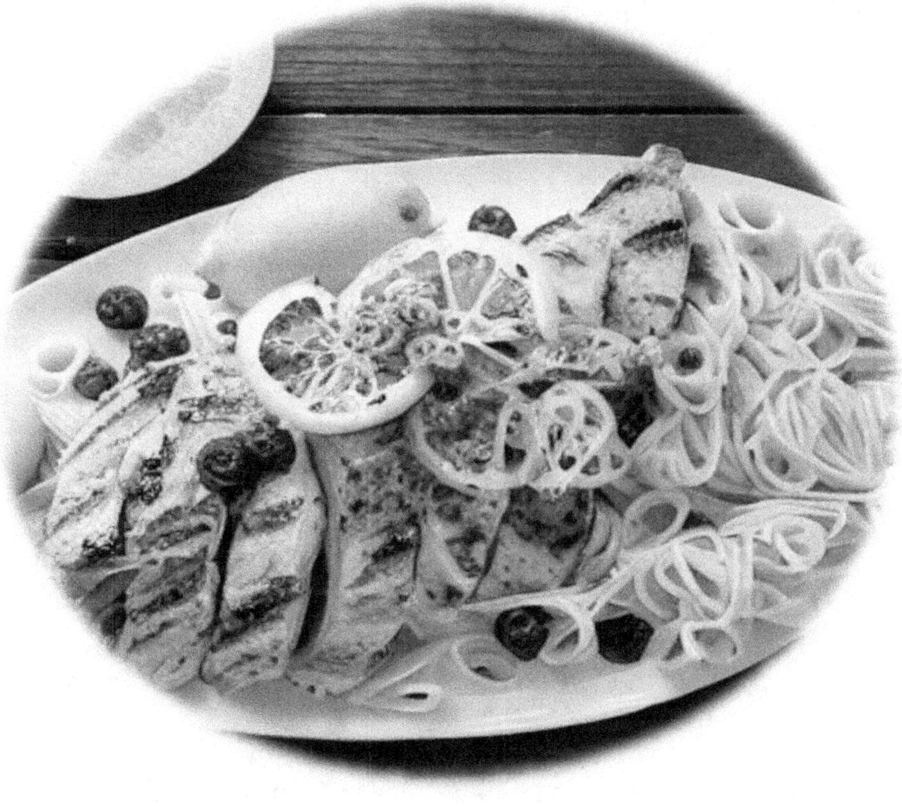

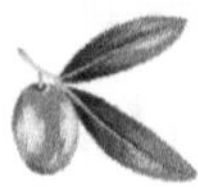

To prepare Mediterranean cuisine at home, it's important to have the right kitchen essentials on hand. Here are some of the key tools and ingredients you'll need:

Olive Oil: Extra-virgin olive oil is a staple of the Mediterranean diet and is used in many recipes for its flavor and health benefits.

Fresh Herbs: Fresh herbs like parsley, basil, oregano, and thyme are commonly used in Mediterranean cooking to add flavor and aroma to dishes.

Spices: Mediterranean cuisine relies on a variety of spices, including cumin, coriander, cinnamon, and paprika, to add depth and complexity to dishes.

Garlic: Garlic is a flavor powerhouse in Mediterranean cooking and is used in many recipes to add depth and aroma to dishes.

Lemon: Lemon juice and zest are used in many Mediterranean recipes to add brightness and acidity to dishes.

Grains: Whole grains like quinoa, farro, and bulgur are commonly used in Mediterranean cuisine to add texture and nutrition to dishes.

Legumes: Legumes like chickpeas, lentils, and beans are a great source of protein and fiber and are used in many Mediterranean recipes, including salads and stews.

Seafood: Seafood is a key component of the Mediterranean diet and is used in many recipes, including grilled fish and seafood stews.

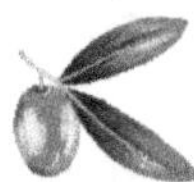

Meats: While meats are consumed in moderation in the Mediterranean diet, lean proteins like chicken and turkey are often used in recipes.

Cooking Utensils: To prepare Mediterranean cuisine, you'll need basic cooking utensils like a chef's knife, cutting board, mixing bowls, and pots and pans.

By having these kitchen essentials on hand, you'll be able to prepare a variety of delicious and healthy Mediterranean meals at home.

Tips for selecting and storing fresh produce

Here are some tips for selecting and storing fresh produce:

Look for Freshness: When shopping for produce, look for items that are firm, plump, and free of bruises or blemishes. Avoid produce that is wilted, mushy, or has an off smell.

Buy Seasonally: Buying produce that is in season is not only more flavorful, but it's also more affordable. Look for produce that is grown locally and in season for the best quality.

Store Properly: Proper storage can help extend the shelf life of fresh produce. Store fruits and vegetables in separate containers in the refrigerator, and keep them dry to prevent spoilage.

Use It or Freeze It: Fresh produce can spoil quickly, so it's important to use it as soon as possible. If you have extra produce that you can't use, consider freezing it for later use.

Wash Thoroughly: Before using fresh produce, be sure to wash it thoroughly to remove any dirt, bacteria, or pesticides.

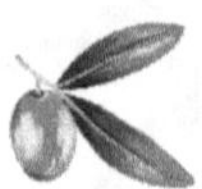

Use a vegetable brush to scrub firm produce like potatoes or carrots.

Eat the Rainbow: To ensure that you're getting a variety of nutrients, try to eat a variety of colorful fruits and vegetables. Aim for at least five servings of fruits and vegetables per day.

By following these tips for selecting and storing fresh produce, you can ensure that you're getting the best quality and nutrition from your fruits and vegetables.

Here are some additional details on selecting and storing fresh produce:

Look for Local and Organic Produce: Local and organic produce is often fresher and more flavorful than produce that has been shipped long distances. Look for farmers' markets or local grocery stores that carry locally-grown produce, and consider choosing organic options when possible.

Check for Ripeness: Different fruits and vegetables have different signs of ripeness. For example, ripe avocados should be firm but give slightly when pressed, while ripe tomatoes should be slightly soft to the touch. Check for signs of ripeness before purchasing to ensure that you're getting the best quality products.

Store at the Right Temperature: Different fruits and vegetables have different ideal storage temperatures. For example, leafy greens and herbs should be stored in the refrigerator at around 32°F to 40°F, while tomatoes and avocados should be stored at room temperature until they are ripe, then refrigerated to extend their shelf life.

Use Fresh Produce Quickly: Fresh produce can spoil quickly, so it's important to use it as soon as possible. Plan your meals around the product you have on hand, and try to use any perishable items within a few days of purchasing.

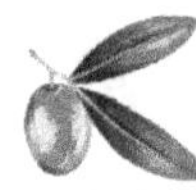

Freeze Extra Produce: If you have extra produce that you can't use in time, consider freezing it for later use. Many fruits and vegetables can be frozen for later use in smoothies, soups, or stir-fries.

Store Fruits and Vegetables Separately: Some fruits and vegetables, such as apples and bananas, produce a gas called ethylene that can cause other produce to ripen and spoil more quickly. To prevent this, store fruits and vegetables in separate containers in the refrigerator.

By following these tips for selecting and storing fresh produce, you can ensure that you're getting the best quality and nutrition from your fruits and vegetables while minimizing waste and spoilage.

What are some common mistakes people make when storing produce?

Here are some common mistakes people make when storing produce:

Not Separating Fruits and Vegetables: As I mentioned earlier, some fruits and vegetables produce ethylene gas, which can cause other produce to ripen and spoil more quickly. It's important to store fruits and vegetables in separate containers in the refrigerator to prevent this.

Storing Produce in Plastic Bags: Storing produce in plastic bags can trap moisture and cause it to spoil more quickly. Instead, store produce in breathable containers or reusable produce bags.

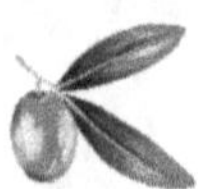

Washing Produce Before Storing: Washing produce before storing can cause it to spoil more quickly. Instead, wait to wash produce until just before using it.

Storing Produce at the Wrong Temperature: Different fruits and vegetables have different ideal storage temperatures. Be sure to store produce at the correct temperature to ensure that it stays fresh as long as possible.

Not Using Produce in Time: Fresh produce can spoil quickly, so it's important to use it as soon as possible. Plan your meals around the product you have on hand, and try to use any perishable items within a few days of purchasing.

Not Freezing Extra Produce: If you have extra produce that you can't use in time, consider freezing it for later use. Many fruits and vegetables can be frozen for later use in smoothies, soups, or stir-fries.

By avoiding these common mistakes when storing produce, you can help ensure that your fruits and vegetables stay fresh and flavorful for as long as possible.

What are some tips for freezing produce?

Here are some helpful tips for freezing produce:

Blanch Before Freezing: Blanching (briefly boiling and then shocking in ice water) is a process that can help preserve the color, texture, and flavor of many fruits and vegetables. Blanching stops the enzymes that cause produce to ripen and break down, which can help maintain its quality during freezing.

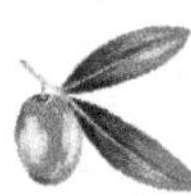

Use High-Quality Produce: High-quality, fresh produce will freeze better than produce that is past its prime. Choose fruits and vegetables that are firm, ripe, and free of blemishes or bruises.

Prepare Produce for Freezing: Before freezing, wash and dry your produce thoroughly. Cut it into pieces or slices if desired, and remove any stems, seeds, or tough skins.

Use Air-Tight Containers: Use air-tight containers or freezer bags to prevent freezer burn and keep produce fresh. Be sure to label the containers with the name of the product and the date it was frozen.

Freeze in Small Portions: Freezing produce in small portions can make it easier to thaw and use later. Consider freezing in portions that are appropriate for the recipes you plan to make.

Use Frozen Produce Within 6 Months: While many fruits and vegetables can be frozen for up to a year, it's best to use them within 6 months for optimal quality.

By following these tips for freezing produce, you can preserve the flavor and nutrition of your favorite fruits and vegetables for later use.

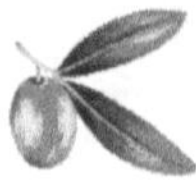

Chapter 3

Appetizers and Snacks

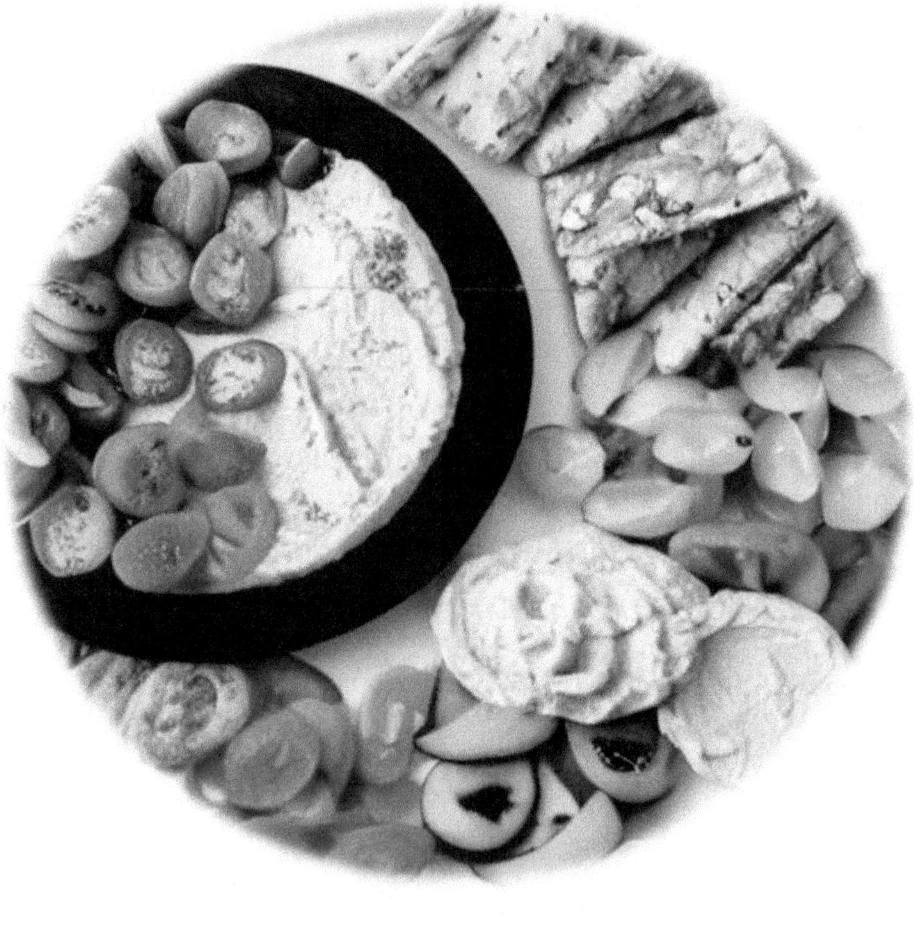

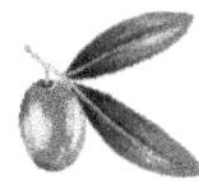

 Here are some delicious and healthy Mediterranean-inspired appetizers and snacks:

Hummus and Veggie Sticks: Serve a bowl of homemade or store-bought hummus with sliced cucumber, bell pepper, and carrot sticks for a healthy and flavorful snack.

Greek Salad Skewers: Thread cherry tomatoes, cucumber, feta cheese, and kalamata olives onto skewers for a colorful and tasty appetizer.

Baba Ganoush: This roasted eggplant dip is similar to hummus and is a great dip for pita bread or veggies. Simply roast eggplant until tender, blend with tahini, lemon juice, garlic, and olive oil, and season with salt and pepper to taste.

Stuffed Grape Leaves: These stuffed grape leaves, also known as dolmas, are a classic Mediterranean appetizer. Fill grape leaves with a mixture of rice, herbs, and spices, and serve with a lemony yogurt sauce.

Roasted Red Pepper and Feta Dip: Roast red peppers until tender, blend with feta cheese, garlic, olive oil, and lemon juice, and season with salt and pepper to taste. Serve with pita bread or veggie sticks.

Spiced Nuts: Toss mixed nuts with a blend of Mediterranean spices like cumin, paprika, and coriander, and roast until crispy and fragrant.

Greek Yogurt and Fruit: Serve a bowl of Greek yogurt topped with fresh fruit like berries, sliced peaches, or chopped figs for a healthy and satisfying snack.

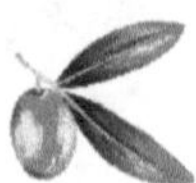

These appetizers and snacks are easy to prepare, packed with flavor and nutrition, and perfect for sharing with friends and family.

----------------/Here are some recipes for flavorful and healthy Mediterranean-inspired appetizers and snacks:

*** Hummus ***

Ingredients:

- 1 can (15 oz) chickpeas, drained and rinsed
- 1/4 cup tahini
- 1/4 cup lemon juice
- 2 cloves garlic, minced
- 1/4 cup olive oil
- Salt and pepper to taste

Instructions:

01- In a food processor, combine the chickpeas, tahini, lemon juice, and garlic.

02- Pulse until smooth, scraping down the sides of the bowl as needed.

03- With the motor running, slowly add the olive oil and process until the hummus is creamy.

04- Season with salt and pepper to taste.

05- Serve with pita bread, veggies, or crackers.

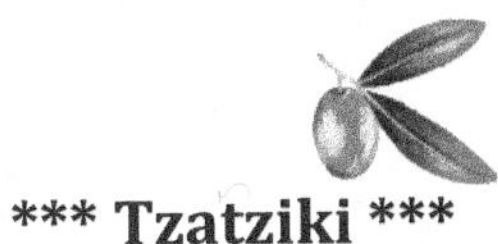

*** Tzatziki ***

Ingredients:

- 1 cup plain Greek yogurt
- 1/2 cup grated cucumber, squeezed of excess liquid
- 1 clove garlic, minced
- 1 tbsp lemon juice
- 1 tbsp chopped fresh dill
- Salt and pepper to taste

Instructions:

01- In a bowl, combine the Greek yogurt, grated cucumber, garlic, lemon juice, and dill.

02-Season with salt and pepper to taste.

03- Chill in the refrigerator for at least 30 minutes before serving.

04- Serve with pita bread, veggies, or grilled meats.

*** Stuffed Grape Leaves (Dolmas)***

Ingredients:

- 1 jar of grape leaves
- 1 cup cooked long-grain rice
- 1/4 cup chopped fresh parsley
- 1/4 cup chopped fresh mint
- 1/4 cup chopped onion

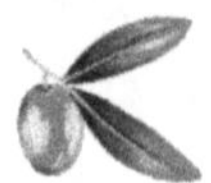

- 2 tbsp lemon juice
- 2 tbsp olive oil
- Salt and pepper to taste

Instructions:

01- Rinse the grape leaves and separate them.

02- In a bowl, combine the cooked rice, parsley, mint, onion, lemon juice, olive oil, salt, and pepper.

03- Place a spoonful of the rice mixture in the center of each grape leaf.

05- Fold the sides of the leaf over the filling and roll it up tightly.

06-Place the stuffed grape leaves in a pot and cover them with water.

07- Bring to a boil, then reduce the heat and simmer for 30 minutes.

08- Serve warm or cold.

These appetizers and snacks are perfect for entertaining or as a quick bite. They are easy to prepare, packed with flavor and nutrition, and are sure to impress your guests. Enjoy!

suggestions for a main course to pair with these appetizers?

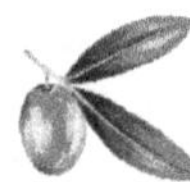

Here are some main course suggestions that would pair well with the Mediterranean-inspired appetizers and snacks:

Grilled Chicken or Fish: Grilled chicken or fish is a great option for a main course that's packed with protein and pairs well with the bright flavors of Mediterranean cuisine. Serve with a side of roasted or grilled vegetables for a complete meal.

Mediterranean Salad: A hearty Mediterranean salad filled with fresh greens, tomatoes, cucumbers, olives, feta cheese, and a lemony vinaigrette is a healthy and satisfying main course option that complements the flavors of the appetizers and snacks.

Vegetable Stew or Ratatouille: A hearty vegetable stew or ratatouille made with eggplant, zucchini, tomatoes, and herbs is a flavorful and filling main course that's perfect for cooler weather.

Lamb or Beef Kebabs: Grilled lamb or beef kebabs are a classic Mediterranean dish that pairs well with the flavors of appetizers and snacks. Serve with a side of rice pilaf or grilled vegetables.

Shakshuka: This popular Middle Eastern dish made with eggs, tomatoes, onions, and spices is a flavorful and satisfying main course option that's perfect for any time of day.

These main course options are easy to prepare and packed with flavor and nutrition, making them the perfect complement to your Mediterranean-inspired appetizers and snacks. Enjoy!

A good recipe for a Mediterranean salad?

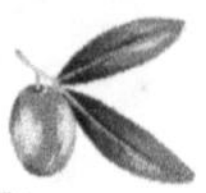

Here's a recipe for a delicious Mediterranean salad:

*** For the Salad ***

Ingredients:

- 6 cups mixed greens
- 1 cup cherry tomatoes, halved
- 1 English cucumber, diced
- 1/2 red onion, thinly sliced
- 1/2 cup kalamata olives
- 1/2 cup crumbled feta cheese

For the Dressing:

- 1/4 cup extra-virgin olive oil
- 2 tbsp red wine vinegar
- 1 clove garlic, minced
- 1 tsp dried oregano
- 1/2 tsp Dijon mustard
- Salt and pepper to taste

Instructions:

01- In a large bowl, combine the mixed greens, cherry tomatoes, cucumber, red onion, kalamata olives, and feta cheese.

02- In a small bowl, whisk together the olive oil, red wine vinegar, garlic, oregano, Dijon mustard, salt, and pepper until well combined.

03- Drizzle the dressing over the salad and toss to coat.

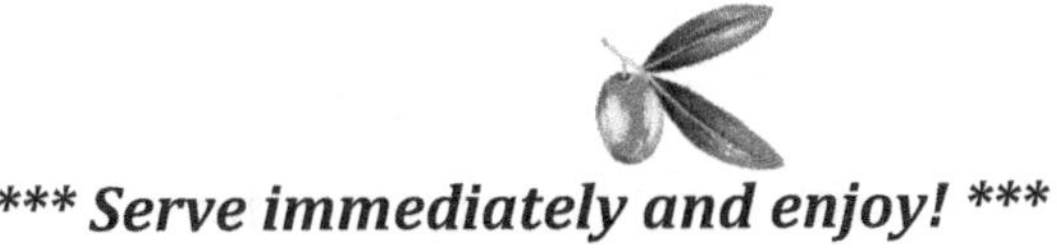

You can also add other Mediterranean-inspired ingredients to the salad, such as roasted red peppers, artichoke hearts, or chickpeas, to make it even more flavorful and satisfying.

What other Mediterranean-inspired ingredients can I add to the salad?

There are many other Mediterranean-inspired ingredients you can add to a salad to make it even more flavorful and nutritious. Here are some options:

Roasted Red Peppers: Roasted red peppers add a sweet, smoky flavor to salads and are a great source of **vitamin C.**

Artichoke Hearts: Artichoke hearts are a classic Mediterranean ingredient that adds a unique texture and flavor to salads. They are also a good source of fiber and antioxidants.

Chickpeas: Chickpeas are versatile ingredients that is commonly used in Mediterranean cuisine. They add protein, fiber, and texture to salads.

Sun-Dried Tomatoes: Sun-dried tomatoes are a concentrated source of flavor and add a sweet, tangy taste to salads. They are also a good source of antioxidants.

Grilled Vegetables: Grilled vegetables like zucchini, eggplant, and bell peppers are a delicious addition to salads and add a smoky flavor and texture.

Quinoa: Quinoa is a gluten-free grain that is commonly used in Mediterranean cuisine. It adds protein, fiber, and texture to salads.

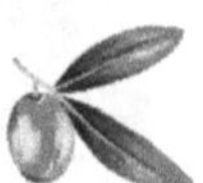

Pine Nuts: Pine nuts are a crunchy and nutty addition to salads and are a good source of healthy fats and protein.

By incorporating these Mediterranean-inspired ingredients into your salads, you can create a delicious and healthy meal that's packed with flavor and nutrition.

some other Mediterranean-inspired dishes I can try?

There are many delicious and healthy Mediterranean-inspired dishes you can try. Here are some ideas:

Greek Moussaka: This classic Greek dish is made with layers of eggplant, ground meat, and a creamy béchamel sauce. It's a hearty and satisfying meal that's perfect for cooler weather.

Chicken Shawarma: Chicken shawarma is a popular Middle Eastern dish that's made with marinated chicken that's grilled or roasted on a spit. Serve with pita bread, hummus, and tzatziki for a complete meal.

Falafel: Falafel is a vegetarian dish made from ground chickpeas, herbs, and spices that are formed into balls and fried until crispy. Serve with pita bread, hummus, and tahini sauce.

Spanakopita: Spanakopita is a Greek dish made with phyllo pastry and a filling of spinach, feta cheese, and herbs. It's a delicious and savory dish that's perfect for entertaining.

Shakshuka: Shakshuka is a Middle Eastern dish that's made with eggs, tomatoes, onions, and spices. It's a flavorful and satisfying dish that's perfect for any time of day.

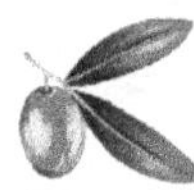

Grilled Fish with Lemon and Herbs: Grilled fish with lemon and herbs is a simple and healthy Mediterranean-inspired dish that's perfect for summer. Serve with a side of grilled vegetables or a Greek salad.

Lentil Soup: Lentil soup is a hearty and nutritious dish that's popular in Mediterranean cuisine. It's made with lentils, vegetables, and herbs and is perfect for cooler weather.

These are just a few examples of the many delicious and healthy Mediterranean-inspired dishes you can try. Experiment with different ingredients and flavors to create your own unique and flavorful meals.

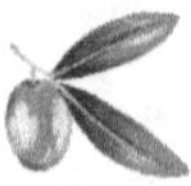

Chapter 4

Soups and Salads

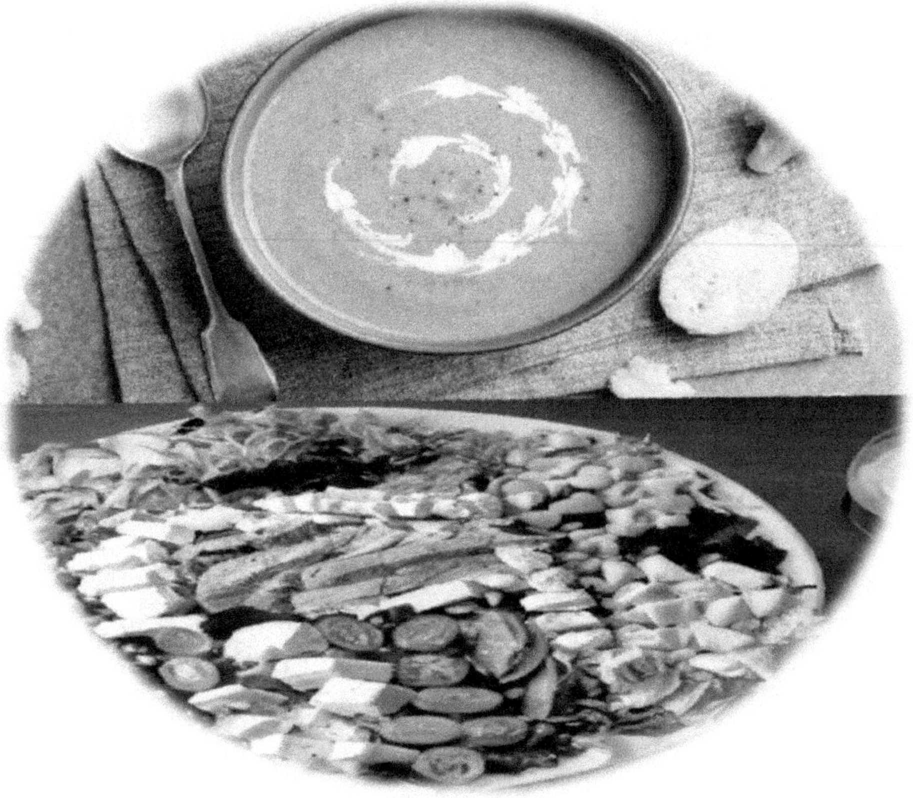

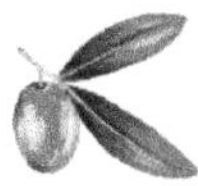

Here are some delicious and healthy Mediterranean-inspired soup and salad recipes:

*** Greek Salad ***

Ingredients:

- 6 cups mixed greens
- 1 cup chopped cucumber
- 1/2 cup cherry tomatoes, halved
- 1/2 cup pitted kalamata olives
- 1/2 cup crumbled feta cheese
- 1/4 cup chopped red onion
- 1/4 cup extra-virgin olive oil
- 2 tbsp red wine vinegar
- 1 tsp dried oregano
- Salt and pepper to taste

Instructions:

01- In a large bowl, combine the mixed greens, cucumber, cherry tomatoes, kalamata olives, feta cheese, and red onion.

02- In a small bowl, whisk together the olive oil, red wine vinegar, oregano, salt, and pepper.

03- Drizzle the dressing over the salad and toss to coat.

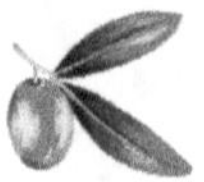

*********Serve immediately and enjoy.*********
34

*** Lentil Sou ***

Ingredients:

- 1 tbsp olive oil
- 1 onion, chopped
- 2 cloves garlic, minced
- 2 carrots, chopped
- 2 celery stalks, chopped
- 1 cup dried lentils, rinsed and drained
- 4 cups vegetable broth
- 1 can (14 oz) diced tomatoes, undrained
- 1 tsp dried thyme
- Salt and pepper to taste

Instructions:

01- In a large pot, heat the olive oil over medium heat.

02- Add the onion and garlic and sauté until the onion is translucent.

03- Add the carrots and celery and continue to sauté for a few more minutes.

04- Add the lentils, vegetable broth, diced tomatoes, thyme, salt, and pepper.

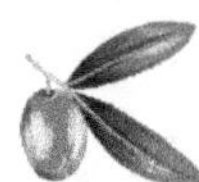

05- Bring the soup to a boil, then reduce the heat and simmer for 30-40 minutes, or until the lentils are tender.

********* *Serve hot and enjoy.*********

*** Fattoush Salad ***

Ingredients

- 6 cups mixed greens
- 1 cup chopped cucumber
- 1 cup cherry tomatoes, halved
- 1/2 cup chopped red onion
- 1/2 cup chopped fresh parsley
- 1/4 cup chopped fresh mint
- 1/4 cup chopped fresh cilantro
- 1/4 cup lemon juice
- 1/4 cup extra-virgin olive oil
- 1 clove garlic, minced
- 1 tsp sumac
- Salt and pepper to taste

Instructions:

01- In a large bowl, combine the mixed greens, cucumber, cherry tomatoes, red onion, parsley, mint, and cilantro.

02- In a small bowl, whisk together the lemon juice, olive oil, garlic, sumac, salt, and pepper.

03- Drizzle the dressing over the salad and toss to coat.

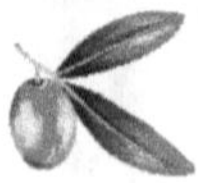

********* **Serve immediately and enjoy.*************

These soup and salad recipes are easy to prepare, packed with flavor and nutrition, and perfect for any time of day.

Vegan soup recipe?

Here's a delicious and healthy vegan Mediterranean-inspired soup recipe:

*** Vegan Chickpea and Vegetable Soup ***

Ingredients:

- 1 tbsp olive oil
- 1 onion, chopped
- 3 cloves garlic, minced
- 2 carrots, chopped
- 2 celery stalks, chopped
- 1 red bell pepper, chopped
- 1 can (15 oz) chickpeas, drained and rinsed
- 1 can (14 oz) diced tomatoes, undrained
- 4 cups vegetable broth
- 1 tsp dried thyme
- 1 tsp ground cumin
- Salt and pepper to taste
- Chopped fresh parsley for garnish

Instructions:

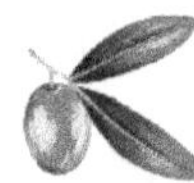

01- In a large pot, heat the olive oil over medium heat.

02- Add the onion and garlic and sauté until the onion is translucent.

03- Add the carrots, celery, and red bell pepper and continue to sauté for a few more minutes.

04- Add the chickpeas, diced tomatoes, vegetable broth, thyme, cumin, salt, and pepper.

05- Bring the soup to a boil, then reduce the heat and simmer for 30-40 minutes, or until the vegetables are tender.

06- Garnish with chopped fresh parsley and serve hot.

This vegan chickpea and vegetable soup is packed with protein, fiber, and flavor, making it a satisfying and healthy meal. It's perfect for a cozy night in or for meal prep for the week ahead.

Other healthy vegan meals

Here are some delicious and healthy vegan meals:

Mediterranean Buddha Bowl: A Buddha bowl is a colorful and nutritious meal that usually consists of a base of grains, topped with veggies, protein, and a flavorful dressing. For a Mediterranean-inspired version, try brown rice or quinoa topped with roasted vegetables like eggplant, zucchini, and bell peppers, chickpeas, hummus, and a lemony tahini dressing.

Falafel Wrap: Falafel is a popular vegan dish made from ground chickpeas, herbs, and spices that are formed into balls and fried until crispy. Wrap the falafel in a whole wheat pita with hummus, chopped veggies, and a drizzle of tahini sauce for a delicious and filling meal.

Lentil Stew: Lentil stew is a hearty and nutritious meal that's easy to prepare. Simply sauté onion, garlic, and spices in a pot, then add lentils, chopped veggies, and vegetable broth. Simmer until the lentils and veggies are tender, then serve with a side of crusty bread.

Vegan Pasta Primavera: Pasta primavera is a classic Italian dish that's perfect for spring and summer. Toss whole wheat pasta with sautéed veggies like bell peppers, zucchini, and cherry tomatoes, then finish with a drizzle of olive oil and a sprinkle of fresh herbs like basil or parsley.

Grilled Portobello Mushroom Burger: Grilled portobello mushrooms make a delicious and satisfying vegan burger. Marinate the mushrooms in balsamic vinegar and olive oil, then grill until tender. Serve on a whole wheat bun with your favorite toppings like avocado, lettuce, and tomato.

These vegan meals are easy to prepare, packed with flavor and nutrition, and perfect for any time of day.

Delicious and healthy vegan desserts:

Fruit Salad: A simple fruit salad is a healthy and refreshing vegan dessert. Combine your favorite fruits like berries, melon, pineapple, and grapes, and serve with a drizzle of maple syrup or a dollop of coconut whipped cream.

Chocolate Avocado Pudding: Avocado makes a creamy and healthy base for vegan pudding. Blend ripe avocado with cocoa powder, almond milk, maple syrup, and vanilla extract

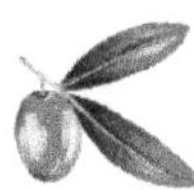

until smooth. Chill in the refrigerator for a few hours, then serve topped with fresh berries or chopped nuts.

Vegan Banana Bread: Banana bread is a classic dessert that's easy to make vegan. Replace the eggs with mashed banana or applesauce, and use plant-based milk and vegan butter. Add in nuts, chocolate chips, or dried fruit for extra flavor and texture.

Chia Seed Pudding: Chia seed pudding is a healthy and protein-packed vegan dessert. Combine chia seeds with almond milk, maple syrup, and vanilla extract, then chill in the refrigerator until thick and creamy. Top with fresh fruit, granola, or nuts.

Vegan Chocolate Chip Cookies: Vegan chocolate chip cookies are a delicious and indulgent dessert. Use vegan butter or coconut oil, and replace the eggs with a flax egg or applesauce. Add in vegan chocolate chips or chunks for a sweet and satisfying treat.

These vegan desserts are easy to prepare, packed with flavor and nutrition, and perfect for any occasion. Enjoy!

Here are some details about each of the vegan desserts I suggested:

Fruit Salad: A fruit salad is a simple and healthy dessert that can be customized to your taste. Choose your favorite fruits and cut them into bite-sized pieces. Drizzle with a little maple syrup, honey, or agave nectar if desired, and serve chilled.

Chocolate Avocado Pudding: Avocado makes a creamy and healthy base for vegan pudding. To make chocolate avocado pudding, blend ripe avocado with cocoa powder, almond milk,

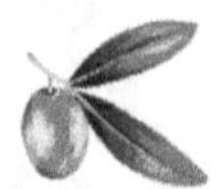

maple syrup, and vanilla extract until smooth. Chill the pudding in the refrigerator for a few hours, then serve topped with fresh berries or chopped nuts.

Vegan Banana Bread: Banana bread is a classic dessert that's easy to make vegan. To make vegan banana bread, replace the eggs with mashed banana or applesauce, and use plant-based milk and vegan butter. Add in nuts, chocolate chips, or dried fruit for extra flavor and texture.

Chia Seed Pudding: Chia seed pudding is a healthy and protein-packed vegan dessert. To make chia seed pudding, combine chia seeds with almond milk, maple syrup, and vanilla extract, then chill in the refrigerator until thick and creamy. Top with fresh fruit, granola, or nuts.

Vegan Chocolate Chip Cookies: Vegan chocolate chip cookies are a delicious and indulgent dessert. To make vegan chocolate chip cookies, use vegan butter or coconut oil, and replace the eggs with a flax egg or applesauce. Add in vegan chocolate chips or chunks for a sweet and satisfying treat.

------ All of these vegan desserts are easy to prepare, packed with flavor and nutrition, and perfect for any occasion. They are also great options if you are looking for healthier dessert alternatives that are free of animal products.

Here are some additional vegan dessert options:

Nice Cream: Nice cream is a healthy and delicious vegan alternative to ice cream. Simply blend frozen bananas with a splash of almond milk until creamy and smooth. Add in other fruits or flavorings like cocoa powder or vanilla extract for additional flavor.

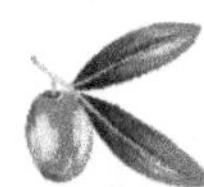

Vegan Cheesecake: Vegan cheesecake is a rich and decadent dessert that's easy to make. Use cashews and coconut cream as the base instead of cream cheese, and sweeten with maple syrup or agave nectar. Top with fresh fruit or a fruit compote for added flavor.

Vegan Tiramisu: Vegan tiramisu is a classic Italian dessert that can be made vegan by using coconut cream instead of mascarpone cheese. Soak ladyfingers in espresso or coffee, then layer with the coconut cream mixture and dust with cocoa powder.

Oatmeal Raisin Cookies: Oatmeal raisin cookies are a classic dessert that can easily be made vegan. Use vegan butter or coconut oil, and replace the eggs with a flax egg or applesauce. Add in rolled oats, raisins, cinnamon, and nutmeg for a delicious and comforting treat.

Vegan Chocolate Mousse: Vegan chocolate mousse is a rich and indulgent dessert that's made with avocado and cocoa powder. Blend ripe avocado with cocoa powder, almond milk, and maple syrup until smooth and creamy. Chill in the refrigerator for a few hours, then serve topped with fresh berries or chopped nuts.

These vegan desserts are all delicious and easy to make. They are perfect for satisfying your sweet tooth while still being healthy and free of animal products.

Vegan substitutes for whipped cream:

There are several vegan substitutes for whipped cream that you can try:

Coconut Whipped Cream: Coconut whipped cream is a popular vegan alternative to traditional whipped cream.

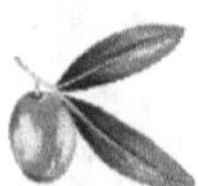

Simply chill a can of full-fat coconut milk in the refrigerator overnight, then scoop out the solid cream that forms on top. Whip the cream with a hand mixer until light and fluffy, then use as you would regular whipped cream.

Aquafaba Whipped Cream: Aquafaba is the liquid from a can of chickpeas or other legumes, and it can be whipped into a foam that's similar in texture to whipped cream. Simply drain a can of chickpeas, then whip the liquid with a hand mixer until it forms stiff peaks. Sweeten with powdered sugar or maple syrup as desired.

Silken Tofu Whipped Cream: Silken tofu can be blended with sweeteners and flavorings to create a creamy and smooth whipped cream substitute. Simply blend silken tofu with vanilla extract, powdered sugar, and a pinch of salt until smooth and fluffy.

Soy Whipped Cream: Soy whipped cream is a vegan alternative to traditional whipped cream that is made with soy milk and other ingredients like coconut oil, sugar, and vanilla extract. It can be found in many stores or made at home using a recipe.

These vegan whipped cream substitutes are all easy to make and delicious. They are perfect for topping fruits, pies, cakes, and other desserts.

Here are some more details about each of the vegan whipped cream substitutes I mentioned:

Coconut Whipped Cream: Coconut whipped cream is a popular vegan alternative to traditional whipped cream. It's made by chilling a can of full-fat coconut milk in the refrigerator overnight, then scooping out the solid cream that forms on top. The cream is then whipped with a hand mixer

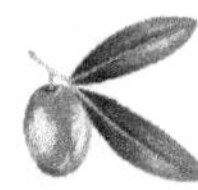

until it forms soft peaks, and sweetened with sugar or other sweeteners as desired. Coconut whipped cream has a slightly sweet and creamy coconut flavor that is perfect for topping fruit, pies, cakes, and other desserts.

Aquafaba Whipped Cream: Aquafaba is the liquid from a can of chickpeas or other legumes, and it can be whipped into a foam that's similar in texture to whipped cream. To make aquafaba whipped cream, simply drain a can of chickpeas and reserve the liquid. Whip the liquid with a hand mixer until it forms stiff peaks, then sweeten with powdered sugar or maple syrup as desired. Aquafaba whipped cream has a light and airy texture that is perfect for topping cakes, pies, and other desserts.

Silken Tofu Whipped Cream: Silken tofu can be blended with sweeteners and flavorings to create a creamy and smooth whipped cream substitute. Simply blend silken tofu with vanilla extract, powdered sugar, and a pinch of salt until smooth and fluffy. Silken tofu whipped cream has a mild and neutral flavor that is perfect for topping fruit, pies, cakes, and other desserts.

Soy Whipped Cream: Soy whipped cream is a vegan alternative to traditional whipped cream that is made with soy milk and other ingredients like coconut oil, sugar, and vanilla extract. It can be found in many stores or made at home using a recipe. Soy whipped cream has a creamy and slightly sweet flavor that is perfect for topping fruit, pies, cakes, and other desserts.

These vegan whipped cream substitutes are all easy to make and delicious. They are perfect for satisfying your sweet tooth while still being healthy and free of animal products.

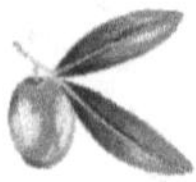

Chapter 5

Main Dishes

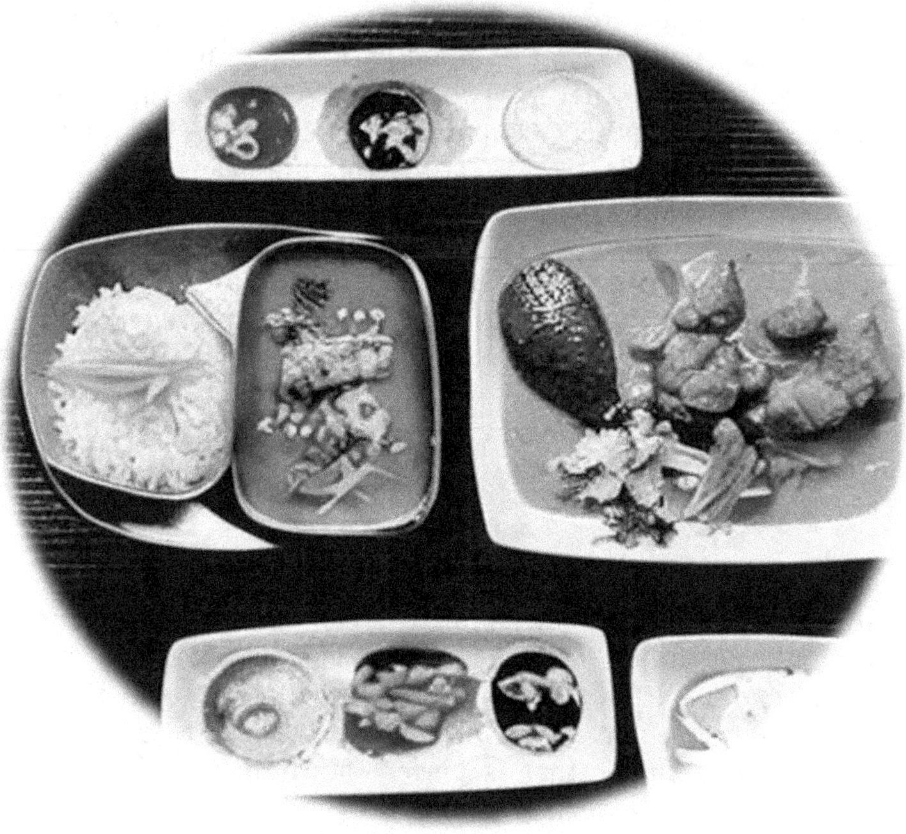

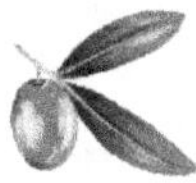

Here are some delicious and healthy Mediterranean-inspired main

*** Grilled Fish ***

Ingredients:

- 4 fresh fish fillets (such as salmon or sea bass)
- 2 tbsp extra-virgin olive oil
- 2 cloves garlic, minced
- 1 tbsp dried oregano
- Salt and pepper to taste
- Lemon wedges for serving

Instructions:

01- Preheat a grill to medium-high heat.

02- In a small bowl, whisk together the olive oil, garlic, oregano, salt, and pepper.

03- Brush the fish fillets with the marinade.

04- Grill the fish for 3-4 minutes per side, or until cooked through.

** Serve with lemon wedges and enjoy.******

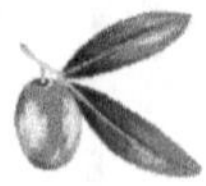

*** Chicken Souvlaki ****

Ingredients:

- 1 lb boneless, skinless chicken breast, cut into chunks
- 1/4 cup extra-virgin olive oil
- 2 cloves garlic, minced
- 1 tbsp dried oregano
- Juice of 1 lemon
- Salt and pepper to taste
- Wooden skewers, soaked in water for 30 minutes

Instructions:

01- In a large bowl, whisk together the olive oil, garlic, oregano, lemon juice, salt, and pepper.

02- Add the chicken chunks to the bowl and toss to coat.

03-Thread the chicken onto the wooden skewers.

04- Preheat a grill to medium-high heat.

05- Grill the chicken skewers for 8-10 minutes, or until cooked through.

**** *Serve hot and enjoy.****

*** Vegetable Lasagna***

Ingredients:

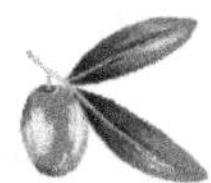

- 9 lasagna noodles, cooked al dente
- 3 cups marinara sauce
- 1 lb zucchini, sliced
- 1 lb yellow squash, sliced
- 1 lb eggplant, sliced
- 2 cups ricotta cheese
- 1/2 cup grated Parmesan cheese
- Salt and pepper to taste
- 2 tbsp chopped fresh basil

Instructions:

01- Preheat the oven to 375°F.

02- Spread 1 cup of marinara sauce in the bottom of a 9x13-inch baking dish.

03- Layer the cooked lasagna noodles on top of the sauce.

04- Arrange the sliced zucchini, yellow squash, and eggplant on top of the noodles.

05- Spoon half of the ricotta cheese on top of the vegetables, then sprinkle with half of the Parmesan cheese and salt and pepper to taste.

06- Repeat the layers with the remaining noodles, vegetables, ricotta cheese, Parmesan cheese, and salt and pepper.

07- Top with the remaining marinara sauce and sprinkle with chopped basil.

08- Cover the dish with foil and bake for 45 minutes.

09- Remove the foil and bake for an additional 10-15 minutes, or until the cheese is melted and bubbly.

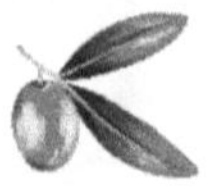

*****Let cool for a few minutes, then serve hot and enjoy.*****

*** Shrimp Scampi ****

Ingredients:

- 1 lb spaghetti
- 2 tbsp extra-virgin olive oil
- 3 cloves garlic, minced
- 1 lb large shrimp, peeled and deveined
- 1/4 cup white wine
- 1/4 cup vegetable broth
- 2 tbsp lemon juice
- Salt and pepper to taste
- 2 tbsp chopped fresh parsley

Instructions:

01- Cook the spaghetti according to the package instructions.

02- In a large skillet, heat the olive oil over medium heat.

03- Add the garlic and sauté for 1-2 minutes, or until fragrant.

04- Add the shrimp to the skillet and sauté for 2-3 minutes, or until pink.

05- Add the white wine, vegetable broth, lemon juice, salt, and pepper to the skillet and simmer for 2-3 minutes.

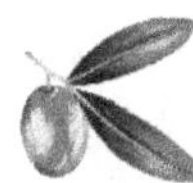

06- Drain the cooked spaghetti and add it to the skillet with the shrimp and sauce.

07- Toss the spaghetti with the shrimp and sauce until well combined.

******* Serve hot and garnish with chopped parsley.********

*** Greek Stuffed Peppers ***

Ingredients:

- 4 bell peppers, halved and seeded
- 1 lb ground beef or lamb
- 1/2 cup uncooked white rice
- 1 onion, chopped
- 2 cloves garlic, minced
- 1 tbsp dried oregano
- 1 tsp dried thyme
- Salt and pepper to taste
- 1 can (14 oz) diced tomatoes
- 1/4 cup chopped fresh parsley

Instructions:

01- Preheat the oven to 375°F.

02- In a large skillet, cook the ground beef or lamb over medium heat until browned.

03- Add the onion, garlic, oregano, thyme, salt, and pepper to the skillet and sauté until the onion is soft.

04- Add the uncooked rice and diced tomatoes to the skillet and stir to combine.

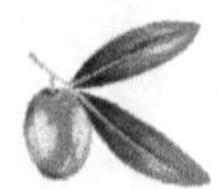

05- Stuff each bell pepper half with the meat and rice mixture.

06- Place the stuffed peppers in a baking dish, cover with foil, and bake for 45 minutes.

07- Remove the foil and bake for an additional 15 minutes, or until the peppers are tender and the filling is cooked through.

**** *Serve hot and garnish with chopped parsley.* ***

*** Ratatouille ***

Ingredients:

- 1 onion, chopped
- 2 cloves garlic, minced
- 1 eggplant, chopped
- 2 zucchini, chopped
- 2 yellow squash, chopped
- 2 bell peppers, chopped
- 1 can (14 oz) diced tomatoes
- 2 tbsp extra-virgin olive oil
- 1 tbsp dried thyme
- Salt and pepper to taste
- 2 tbsp chopped fresh basil

Instructions:

01- Preheat the oven to 375°F.

02- In a large skillet, heat the olive oil over medium heat.

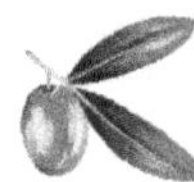

03- Add the onion and garlic to the skillet and sauté until the onion is soft.

04- Add the eggplant, zucchini, yellow squash, and bell peppers to the skillet and sauté until the vegetables are tender.

05- Add the diced tomatoes, thyme, salt, and pepper to the skillet and stir to combine.

06- Transfer the vegetable mixture to a baking dish.

07- Cover the dish with foil and bake for 45 minutes.

08- Remove the foil and bake for an additional 15 minutes, or until the vegetables are cooked through.

Serve hot and garnish with chopped basil.

These Mediterranean-inspired main course recipes are easy to prepare and packed with flavor and nutrition. It's perfect for a family dinner or for entertaining guests.

Here are some additional details about each of the Mediterranean-inspired main dish recipes I suggested:

Grilled Fish: Grilled fish is a healthy and flavorful Mediterranean-inspired main dish that's perfect for summer. For this recipe, you can use any fresh fish fillets, such as salmon or sea bass. The fish is marinated in a mixture of olive oil, garlic, oregano, salt, and pepper, then grilled until cooked

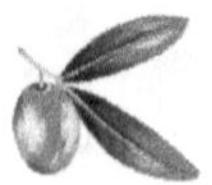

through. Serve with lemon wedges for a bright and citrusy finish.

Chicken Souvlaki: Chicken souvlaki is a classic Greek dish that's easy to prepare and packed with flavor. For this recipe, boneless, skinless chicken breast is cut into chunks and marinated in a mixture of olive oil, garlic, oregano, lemon juice, salt, and pepper. The chicken is then threaded onto wooden skewers and grilled until cooked through. Serve with a side of Greek salad or roasted vegetables for a complete meal.

Vegetable Lasagna: Vegetable lasagna is a healthy and delicious way to enjoy a classic Italian dish. For this recipe, lasagna noodles are layered with sliced zucchini, yellow squash, and eggplant, as well as ricotta cheese and Parmesan cheese. The lasagna is then baked in the oven until the cheese is melted and bubbly. Serve with a side salad or garlic bread for a comforting and satisfying meal.

These Mediterranean-inspired main dish recipes are easy to make and perfect for a family dinner or entertaining guests. They are packed with flavor and nutrition and can be customized to your taste by adding your favorite herbs and spices.

Some healthy side dishes that would complement these main courses:

Here are some healthy side dishes that would complement these Mediterranean-inspired main courses:

Greek Salad: A Greek salad is a classic side dish that's easy to prepare and packed with flavor. Simply toss together chopped lettuce, sliced cucumbers, diced tomatoes, chopped red onion,

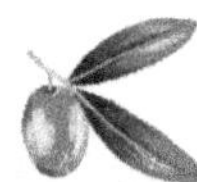

and crumbled feta cheese. Dress with a simple vinaigrette made with olive oil, lemon juice, and oregano.

Roasted Vegetables: Roasted vegetables are a healthy and delicious side dish that pairs well with grilled fish, chicken souvlaki, and vegetable lasagna. Simply toss your favorite vegetables, such as bell peppers, zucchini, eggplant, and cherry tomatoes, with olive oil and seasonings like garlic, oregano, and thyme. Roast in the oven until tender and caramelized.

Tzatziki Sauce: Tzatziki sauce is a creamy and tangy dip that's perfect for serving with grilled chicken souvlaki or shrimp scampi. To make tzatziki, simply mix together plain Greek yogurt, grated cucumber, minced garlic, lemon juice, and chopped fresh dill. Season with salt and pepper to taste.

Quinoa Salad: Quinoa salad is a healthy and filling side dish that's perfect for serving with grilled fish or stuffed peppers. Cook quinoa according to package instructions, then mix with chopped vegetables like bell peppers, cherry tomatoes, and red onion. Dress with a simple vinaigrette made with olive oil, lemon juice, and herbs like parsley and basil.

Grilled Vegetables: Grilled vegetables are a healthy and delicious side dish that pairs well with shrimp scampi or ratatouille. Simply brush sliced vegetables like zucchini, eggplant, and bell peppers with olive oil and grill until tender and caramelized. Season with salt, pepper, and herbs like rosemary or thyme.

These healthy side dishes are easy to prepare and packed with flavor and nutrition. They are perfect for complementing your Mediterranean-inspired main courses and adding variety to your meals.

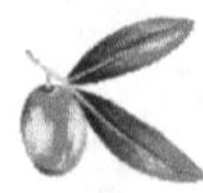

Greek Salad: A Greek salad is a classic Mediterranean side dish that's easy to prepare and packed with flavor. It typically includes chopped lettuce, sliced cucumbers, diced tomatoes, chopped red onion, and crumbled feta cheese. The salad is dressed with a simple vinaigrette made with olive oil, lemon juice, and oregano. You can also add other ingredients like Kalamata olives, bell peppers, and fresh herbs.

Roasted Vegetables: Roasted vegetables are a healthy and delicious side dish that pairs well with a variety of Mediterranean main courses. You can use any vegetables you like, such as bell peppers, zucchini, eggplant, and cherry tomatoes. Simply toss the vegetables with olive oil and seasonings like garlic, oregano, and thyme. Roast in the oven until tender and caramelized. Roasting concentrates the flavors of the vegetables and brings out their natural sweetness.

Tzatziki Sauce: Tzatziki sauce is a creamy and tangy dip that's perfect for serving with grilled chicken souvlaki or shrimp scampi. It's made with plain Greek yogurt, grated cucumber, minced garlic, lemon juice, and chopped fresh dill. The dip is seasoned with salt and pepper to taste. Tzatziki is a refreshing and healthy alternative to heavier dips like ranch or blue cheese.

Quinoa Salad: Quinoa salad is a healthy and filling side dish that's perfect for serving with grilled fish or stuffed peppers. Quinoa is a high-protein grain that's gluten-free and easy to digest. To make the salad, cook quinoa according to package instructions, then mix it with chopped vegetables like bell peppers, cherry tomatoes, and red onion. Dress the salad with

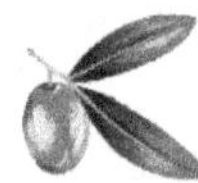

a simple vinaigrette made with olive oil, lemon juice, and herbs like parsley and basil.

Grilled Vegetables: Grilled vegetables are a healthy and delicious side dish that pairs well with shrimp scampi or ratatouille. Grilling vegetables gives them a smoky and charred flavor that's hard to resist. Simply brush sliced vegetables like zucchini, eggplant, and bell peppers with olive oil and grill until tender and caramelized. Season the vegetables with salt, pepper, and herbs like rosemary or thyme.

These healthy side dishes are easy to prepare and perfect for complementing your Mediterranean-inspired main courses. They are packed with fresh flavors, vitamins, and minerals, and can be customized to your taste by adding your favorite herbs and spices.

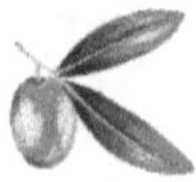

Chapter 6

Sides and Accompaniments

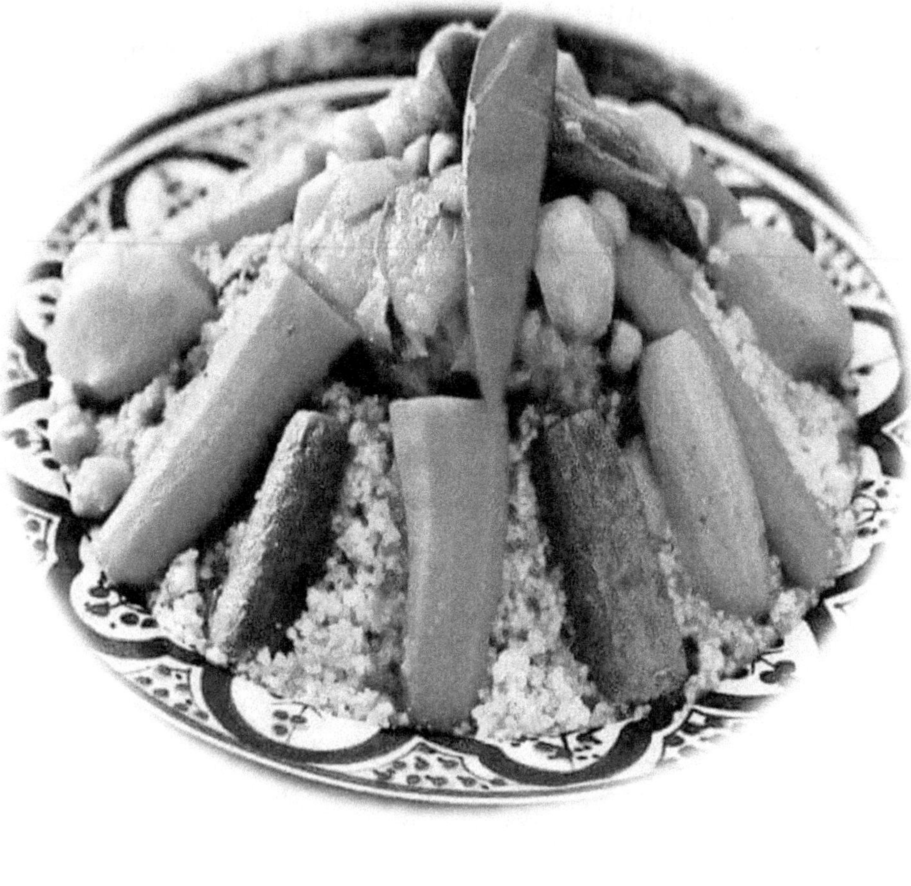

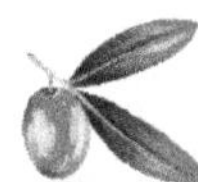

Recipes for healthy and flavorful Mediterranean side dishes, such as roasted vegetables, couscous, and quinoa.

Here are some healthy and flavorful Mediterranean side dish recipes:

*****Roasted Vegetables*****

Ingredients:

- 1 lb mixed vegetables (such as bell peppers, zucchini, eggplant, and cherry tomatoes)
- 2 tbsp extra-virgin olive oil
- 2 cloves garlic, minced
- 1 tbsp dried oregano
- Salt and pepper to taste
- Lemon wedges for serving

Instructions:

01- Preheat the oven to 400°F.

02- Cut the vegetables into bite-sized pieces and place them on a baking sheet.

03- In a small bowl, whisk together the olive oil, garlic, oregano, salt, and pepper.

04- Drizzle the marinade over the vegetables and toss to coat.

05- Roast the vegetables in the oven for 20-25 minutes, or until tender and caramelized.

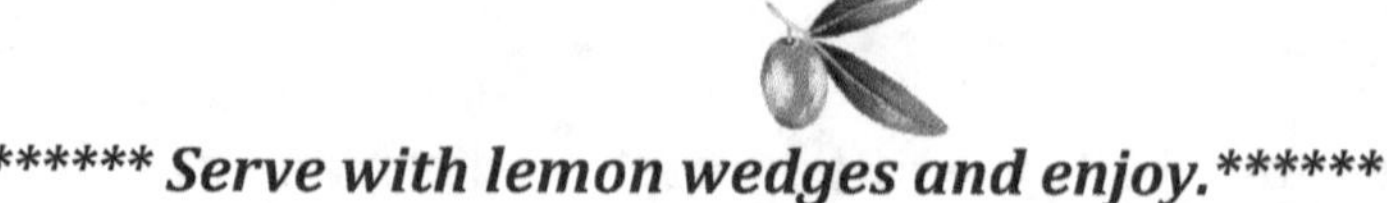

****** Serve with lemon wedges and enjoy.******

****** Couscous Salad *****

Ingredients:

- 1 cup couscous
- 1 1/4 cups vegetable broth
- 1/4 cup extra-virgin olive oil
- 2 tbsp lemon juice
- 1 tsp honey
- 1/2 tsp ground cumin
- Salt and pepper to taste
- 1 cup chopped fresh vegetables (such as cucumbers, tomatoes, and red onion)
- 1/4 cup chopped fresh parsley

Instructions:

01- Bring the vegetable broth to a boil in a small saucepan.

02- Add the couscous to the saucepan, cover, and remove from heat.

03- Let the couscous sit for 5-10 minutes, or until the liquid is absorbed.

04- In a small bowl, whisk together the olive oil, lemon juice, honey, cumin, salt, and pepper.

05- Fluff the couscous with a fork and transfer it to a large bowl.

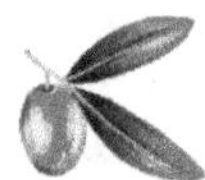

06- Add the chopped vegetables and parsley to the bowl and toss to combine.

07- Pour the dressing over the couscous salad and toss to coat.

**** *Serve chilled or at room temperature and enjoy.* ****

*** Quinoa and Chickpea Salad***

Ingredients:

- 1 cup quinoa
- 2 cups water
- 1 can (14 oz) chickpeas, drained and rinsed
- 1 red bell pepper, chopped
- 1/2 red onion, chopped
- 1/4 cup chopped fresh parsley
- 1/4 cup extra-virgin olive oil
- 2 tbsp lemon juice
- 1 tsp ground cumin
- Salt and pepper to taste

Instructions:

01- Rinse the quinoa under cold water and drain.

02- In a medium saucepan, bring the water to a boil.

03- Add the quinoa to the saucepan, cover, and reduce heat to low.

04- Simmer the quinoa for 15-20 minutes, or until the liquid is absorbed.

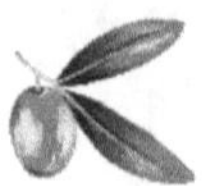

05- In a large bowl, combine the cooked quinoa, chickpeas, bell pepper, red onion, and parsley.

06- In a small bowl, whisk together the olive oil, lemon juice, cumin, salt, and pepper.

07- Pour the dressing over the quinoa salad and toss to coat.

****** *Serve chilled or at room temperature and enjoy*****

These healthy and flavorful Mediterranean side dish recipes are easy to prepare and perfect for complementing your main courses. They are packed with fresh flavors, vitamins, and minerals, and can be customized to your taste by adding your favorite herbs and spices.

Tips for making roasted vegetables more flavorful

Here are some tips for making your roasted vegetables more flavorful:

Use a variety of vegetables: Mix and match different vegetables to add variety and texture to your roasted vegetables. Try using a combination of bell peppers, zucchini, eggplant, cherry tomatoes, onions, and mushrooms.

Add fresh herbs: Fresh herbs like rosemary, thyme, and oregano add a burst of flavor to roasted vegetables. Simply chop the herbs and sprinkle them over the vegetables before roasting.

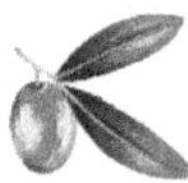

Use garlic and onions: Garlic and onions are both great flavor boosters for roasted vegetables. Toss them with the vegetables before roasting them to infuse them with flavor.

Add some spice: Spices like cumin, paprika, and chili powder can add a kick of flavor to roasted vegetables. Sprinkle them over the vegetables before roasting them for added depth of flavor.

Use high-quality olive oil: A good quality extra-virgin olive oil can add richness and depth of flavor to roasted vegetables. Drizzle the vegetables with olive oil before roasting and toss to coat.

Don't overcrowd the pan: Make sure to spread the vegetables out in a single layer on the baking sheet. Overcrowding the pan can lead to steaming instead of roasting, which can result in soggy vegetables.

By following these tips, you can make your roasted vegetables more flavorful and delicious.

Use balsamic vinegar to add flavor to roasted vegetables.

Yes, you can use balsamic vinegar to add flavor to roasted vegetables. Balsamic vinegar is a great way to add a tangy and slightly sweet flavor to roasted vegetables. Simply drizzle the vegetables with balsamic vinegar before roasting, or toss them with the vinegar after they come out of the oven. Here's a simple recipe for roasted vegetables with balsamic vinegar:

Ingredients:

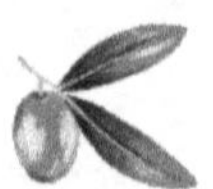

- 1 lb mixed vegetables (such as bell peppers, zucchini, eggplant, and cherry tomatoes)
- 2 tbsp extra-virgin olive oil
- 2 cloves garlic, minced
- Salt and pepper to taste
- 2 tbsp balsamic vinegar

Instructions:

01- Preheat the oven to 400°F.

02- Cut the vegetables into bite-sized pieces and place them on a baking sheet.

03- In a small bowl, whisk together the olive oil, garlic, salt, and pepper.

04- Drizzle the marinade over the vegetables and toss to coat.

05- Roast the vegetables in the oven for 20-25 minutes, or until tender and caramelized.

06- Drizzle the roasted vegetables with balsamic vinegar and toss to coat.

Adding balsamic vinegar to your roasted vegetables is a simple and delicious way to enhance their flavor. However, be sure to use the vinegar in moderation, as a little goes a long way.

Some other ways to add flavor to roasted vegetables

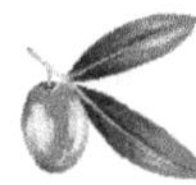

Here are some other ways to add flavor to roasted vegetables:

Use different cooking oils: Instead of using olive oil, try using other oils like sesame oil or coconut oil to add a different flavor to your roasted vegetables. Different oils have different flavor profiles and can add a unique taste to your dish.

Try different kinds of vinegar: Balsamic vinegar is a popular choice for roasted vegetables, but other types of vinegar can also add flavor. Apple cider vinegar and rice vinegar are all great options to try.

Add citrus: Squeeze fresh lemon or lime juice over your roasted vegetables for a bright, zesty flavor. Citrus can also add a touch of acidity that balances out the sweetness of roasted vegetables.

Add cheese: Sprinkle-grated Parmesan, feta, or goat cheese over your roasted vegetables for a rich, savory flavor. Cheese can also add a creamy texture to your dish.

Use spice blends: Experiment with different spice blends to add flavor to your roasted vegetables. Za'atar, curry powder, and garam masala are all great options to try.

Add nuts or seeds: Toasted nuts or seeds like pine nuts, almonds, or sesame seeds can add a crunchy texture and nutty flavor to your roasted vegetables.

By using different oils, vinegar, spices, and toppings, you can add a variety of flavors and textures to your roasted vegetables. Don't be afraid to experiment and try new flavor combinations to find your favorite.

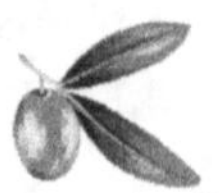

Nuts and seeds that pair well with roasted vegetables

Here are some nuts and seeds that pair well with roasted vegetables:

Almonds: Almonds add a crunchy texture and nutty flavor to roasted vegetables. They pair well with vegetables such as Brussels sprouts, carrots, and butternut squash.

Pine nuts: Pine nuts are small and fluffy, with a buttery texture and nutty flavor. It pairs well with roasted vegetables such as eggplant, zucchini, and cherry tomatoes.

Nuts: Nuts are rich and earthy, with a slightly bitter flavor. They pair well with roasted vegetables such as beets, sweet potatoes, and Brussels sprouts.

Pistachios: Pistachios are slightly sweet, nutty, and have a light green color that adds visual interest to roasted vegetables. It pairs well with vegetables such as broccoli, carrots, and bell peppers.

Sesame Seeds: Sesame seeds have a nutty flavor and add a subtle crunch to roasted vegetables. They pair well with vegetables such as broccoli, green beans, and asparagus.

Sunflower Seeds: Sunflower seeds have a nutty flavor and a slightly crunchy texture. It pairs well with roasted vegetables such as butternut squash, sweet potatoes, and carrots.

By adding nuts or seeds to roasted vegetables, you can add a crunchy texture and boost nutrition. They also add flavor and interest to your dish. Experiment with different types of nuts and seeds to find your favorite combination.

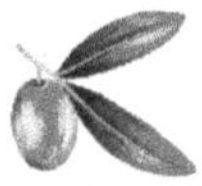

Chapter 7

Desserts and Sweets

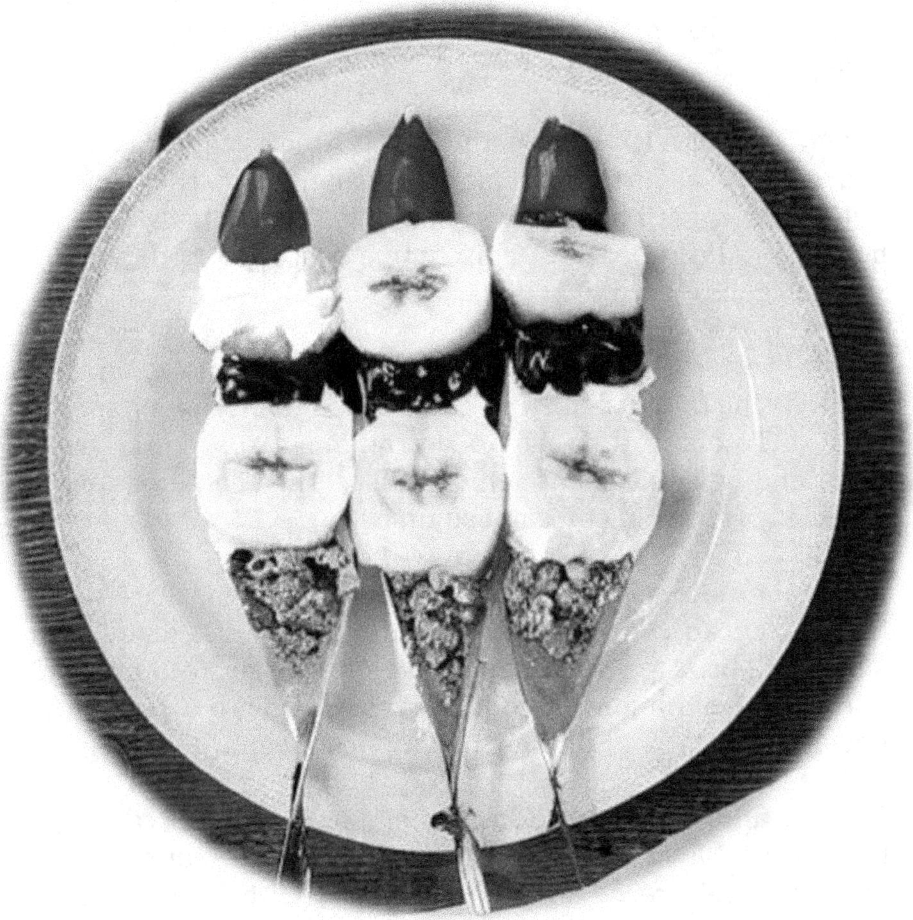

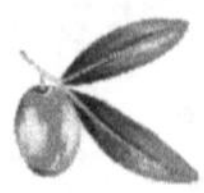

Mediterranean desserts and sweets are inspired by the traditional flavors and ingredients of the Mediterranean region. They are often made with natural and wholesome ingredients like fresh fruit, nuts, honey, and olive oil, and are lower in sugar and unhealthy fats than many Western desserts. Here are some examples of Mediterranean desserts and sweets:

Greek Yogurt with Honey and Fruit: Greek yogurt is a thick and creamy yogurt that's high in protein and calcium. It's often served with a drizzle of honey and fresh fruit, such as berries or sliced peaches. This simple dessert is both healthy and delicious.

Fresh Fruit with Mint and Lemon: Fresh fruit is a staple in Mediterranean cuisine, and is often served as a simple dessert. To elevate the flavors, try adding a sprinkle of fresh mint and a squeeze of lemon juice. This combination is especially refreshing on a hot summer day.

Almond Cake: Almond cake is a popular dessert in Mediterranean countries like Spain and Italy. It's made with almond flour, eggs, sugar, and olive oil, and has a moist and nutty texture. Almond cake is often served with a dusting of powdered sugar and a dollop of whipped cream.

Orange and Olive Oil Cake: Orange and olive oil cake is a moist and flavorful cake that's popular in Mediterranean countries like Greece and Italy. It's made with olive oil, fresh oranges, flour, and sugar, and has a light and citrusy flavor. Orange and olive oil cake is often served with a drizzle of honey or a sprinkle of powdered sugar.

Baklava: Baklava is a sweet and flaky pastry that's popular in Mediterranean and Middle Eastern cuisine. It's made with layers of phyllo dough, chopped nuts, and a sweet syrup made

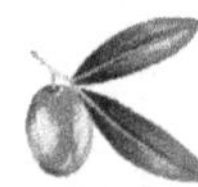

with honey, sugar, and cinnamon. Baklava is a labor of love, but the end result is a delicious and impressive dessert that's perfect for special occasions.

Mediterranean desserts and sweets are a great way to satisfy your sweet tooth while still sticking to a healthy and balanced diet. They use natural and wholesome ingredients and are often lower in sugar and unhealthy fats than many Western desserts.

Sweet treats that are inspired by the Mediterranean diet. Recipes will include baklava, fruit sorbet, and almond cookies.

Here are some sweet treats inspired by the Mediterranean diet:

*** Baklava ***

Ingredients:

- 1 lb phyllo dough
- 1 1/2 cups chopped nuts (such as walnuts, pistachios, or almonds)
- 1/2 cup honey
- 1/2 cup water
- 1/2 cup unsalted butter, melted
- 1 tsp ground cinnamon

Instructions:

01- Preheat the oven to 350°F.

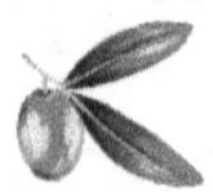

02- In a small saucepan, combine the honey, water, and cinnamon. Bring to a boil and simmer for 5 minutes.

03- Remove the saucepan from the heat and let the syrup cool.

04- Brush a 9x13-inch baking dish with melted butter.

05-Lay a sheet of phyllo dough in the bottom of the dish and brush it with melted butter.

06- Repeat with 7-8 sheets of phyllo dough, brushing each sheet with melted butter.

07- Sprinkle the chopped nuts over the phyllo dough.

08- Layer 7-8 more sheets of phyllo dough on top of the nuts, brushing each sheet with melted butter.

09- Use a sharp knife to cut the baklava into small diamond shapes.

10- Bake the baklava in the oven for 30-35 minutes, or until golden brown.

11- Remove the baklava from the oven and pour the cooled syrup over the top.

12- Let the baklava cool before serving.

****** Fruit Sorbet ******

Ingredients:

- 4 cups fresh fruit (such as strawberries, raspberries, or mango)

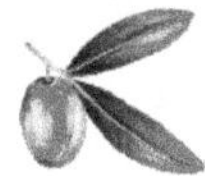

- 1 cup water
- 1 cup sugar
- 2 tbsp lemon juice

Instructions:

01- Puree the fresh fruit in a blender or food processor.

02- In a small saucepan, combine the water and sugar. Bring to a boil and simmer for 5 minutes.

03- Remove the saucepan from the heat and let the syrup cool.

04- Add the cooled syrup and lemon juice to the fruit puree and pulse until combined.

05- Pour the mixture into a shallow dish and freeze for 2-3 hours, or until solid.

06- Use a fork to scrape the sorbet into small crystals.

07- Freeze the sorbet for another 1-2 hours, or until firm.

*** Almond Cookies ***

Ingredients:

- 2 cups almond flour
- 1/2 cup honey
- 1/2 cup unsalted butter, melted
- 1 tsp vanilla extract
- 1/4 tsp salt

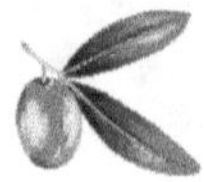

Instructions:

01- Preheat the oven to 350°F.

02- In a large bowl, mix together the almond flour, honey, melted butter, vanilla extract, and salt.

03- Use a cookie scoop or spoon to drop the dough onto a baking sheet lined with parchment paper.

04- Flatten each cookie slightly with the back of a fork.

05- Bake the cookies in the oven for 10-12 minutes, or until golden brown.

06- Let the cookies cool before serving.

These sweet treats inspired by the Mediterranean diet are delicious and easy to make. They use natural and wholesome ingredients like fresh fruit, nuts, and honey, and are perfect for satisfying your sweet tooth while still sticking with a healthy eating plan.

Here is some more information about each of the Mediterranean-inspired sweet treats:

Baklava: Baklava is a sweet and flaky pastry that's popular in Mediterranean cuisine. It's made with layers of phyllo dough, chopped nuts, and a sweet syrup made with honey, sugar, and cinnamon. The phyllo dough is brushed with melted butter to create a crispy, golden crust. Baklava is a labor of love, but the end result is a delicious and impressive dessert that's perfect for special occasions.

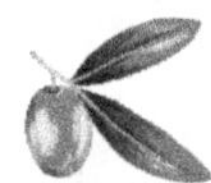

Fruit Sorbet: Fruit sorbet is a refreshing and healthy dessert that's perfect for hot summer days. It's made with fresh fruit, water, sugar, and lemon juice. The mixture is pureed in a blender or food processor, then frozen until solid. The sorbet is then scraped into small crystals and frozen again until firm. Fruit sorbet is a great alternative to ice cream, as it's lower in fat and calories and higher in vitamins and antioxidants.

Almond Cookies: Almond cookies are a sweet and nutty treat that's perfect for snacking or dessert. They're made with almond flour, honey, melted butter, vanilla extract, and salt. The dough is dropped onto a baking sheet and flattened with a fork before baking. Almond cookies are gluten-free and naturally sweetened, making them a healthier alternative to traditional cookies.

These Mediterranean-inspired sweet treats are easy to make and use natural and wholesome ingredients. They're perfect for satisfying your sweet tooth while still sticking with a healthy eating plan.

Other popular Mediterranean desserts

Here are some other popular Mediterranean desserts:

Tiramisu: Tiramisu is an Italian dessert made with ladyfingers, espresso, mascarpone cheese, and cocoa powder. It has a creamy and rich flavor and is often dusted with cocoa powder or grated chocolate.

Semolina Halva: Semolina halva is a traditional Greek dessert made with semolina flour, sugar, water, and butter. It has a dense and crumbly texture and is often flavored with cinnamon, cloves, or orange zest.

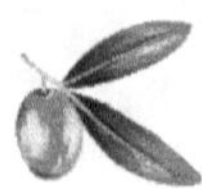

Pastel de Nata: Pastel de nata is a Portuguese egg tart pastry that's made with a flaky pastry crust and a creamy custard filling. It's often sprinkled with cinnamon and powdered sugar.

Kanafeh: Kanafeh is a Middle Eastern dessert made with shredded phyllo dough, cheese, and a sweet syrup made with sugar and rose water. It has a crispy and chewy texture and is often topped with chopped pistachios.

Sfogliatelle: Sfogliatelle is an Italian pastry that's made with layers of flaky dough and a sweet ricotta filling. It has a crispy and buttery texture and is often dusted with powdered sugar.

These Mediterranean desserts are all delicious and made with natural and wholesome ingredients. They're often lower in sugar and unhealthy fats than many Western desserts, making them a healthier and more nutritious option

Which of these desserts is the easiest to make at home?

Greek Yogurt with Honey and Fruit are the easiest to make at home among the Mediterranean desserts mentioned. All you need is a cup of Greek yogurt, fresh fruit, and honey. Simply spoon some Greek yogurt into a bowl, top with fresh fruit, and drizzle with honey. You can also add some chopped nuts or granola for extra crunch. It's a simple and healthy dessert that can be made in minutes with minimal effort.

Greek yogurt with honey and fruit is not only easy to make, but it's also a healthy and nutritious dessert option. Greek yogurt is a good source of protein and calcium, and it's lower

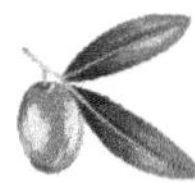

in sugar and fat than many other types of yogurt. It's also thick and creamy, which makes it a great base for desserts.

To make this dessert, simply choose your favorite fresh fruit, such as berries, peaches, or bananas, and chop it into bite-sized pieces. Spoon some Greek yogurt into a bowl, and top it with the fruit. Drizzle honey over the top to add sweetness and flavor.

You can also get creative with your toppings. Try adding chopped nuts, like almonds or walnuts, for some crunch, or sprinkle some granola over the top for added texture. You can also add a sprinkle of cinnamon or a squeeze of lemon juice for extra flavor.

Greek yogurt with honey and fruit is a simple and satisfying dessert that's easy to make at home. It's a great way to satisfy your sweet tooth while still sticking to a healthy eating plan.

Other healthy dessert options

Here are some other healthy dessert options you can try:

Fresh Fruit Salad: A fruit salad is a simple and refreshing dessert that's naturally sweet and packed with vitamins and antioxidants. You can mix and match your favorite fruits, such as berries, melons, kiwis, and citrus, for a colorful and delicious dessert.

Chia Seed Pudding: Chia seed pudding is a nutritious and creamy dessert that's made with chia seeds, milk, and sweetener. Chia seeds are high in fiber and omega-3 fatty acids, and they absorb liquid to create a pudding-like consistency. You can add flavors like vanilla, chocolate, or fruit to customize your pudding.

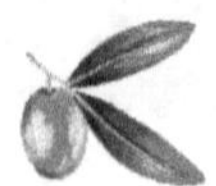

Baked Apples: Baked apples are a warm and comforting dessert that's easy to make. Simply core an apple and fill it with a mixture of oats, cinnamon, and honey. Bake in the oven until tender and serve with a dollop of Greek yogurt or whipped cream.

Dark Chocolate: Dark chocolate is a rich and indulgent dessert that's also high in antioxidants and flavonoids. Choose dark chocolate with at least 70% cacao for the most health benefits, and enjoy a small piece or two as a treat.

Frozen Yogurt Bark: Frozen yogurt bark is a fun and colorful dessert that's made by spreading Greek yogurt on a baking sheet and topping it with fresh fruit, nuts, and granola. Freeze until firm, then break into pieces and serve.

These healthy dessert options are all delicious and satisfying, and they use natural and wholesome ingredients. They're a great way to satisfy your sweet tooth while still sticking to a healthy eating plan.

Here's some more information on each of the healthy dessert options:

Fresh Fruit Salad: Fresh fruit salad is a simple and refreshing dessert that's perfect for summer. Fresh fruit is naturally sweet and high in vitamins and antioxidants, making it a healthy and nutritious dessert option. You can mix and match your favorite fruits, and add a squeeze of lemon juice or a sprinkle of mint for extra flavor.

Chia Seed Pudding: Chia seed pudding is a creamy and satisfying dessert that's high in fiber, protein, and omega-3 fatty acids. Chia seeds absorb liquid to create a pudding-like

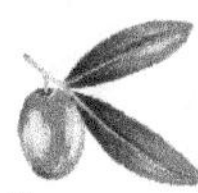

consistency, and they can be flavored with a variety of ingredients like vanilla extract, cocoa powder, or fruit. Chia seed pudding is a great alternative to traditional pudding or custard, as it's lower in sugar and fat.

Baked Apples: Baked apples are a warm and comforting dessert that's easy to make. Simply core an apple and fill it with a mixture of oats, cinnamon, and honey. Bake in the oven until tender and serve with a dollop of Greek yogurt or whipped cream. Baked apples are a healthier alternative to apple pie or crumble, as they're lower in sugar and fat.

Dark Chocolate: Dark chocolate is a rich and indulgent dessert that's also high in antioxidants and flavonoids. Choose dark chocolate with at least 70% cacao for the most health benefits, and enjoy a small piece or two as a treat. Dark chocolate is a great alternative to milk chocolate or candy, as it's lower in sugar and higher in nutrients.

Frozen Yogurt Bark: Frozen yogurt bark is a fun and colorful dessert that's made by spreading Greek yogurt on a baking sheet and topping it with fresh fruit, nuts, and granola. Freeze until firm, then break into pieces and serve. Frozen yogurt bark is a healthier alternative to ice cream or candy, as it's lower in sugar and higher in protein.

These healthy dessert options are all delicious and satisfying, and they use natural and wholesome ingredients. They're a great way to satisfy your sweet tooth while still sticking to a healthy eating plan.

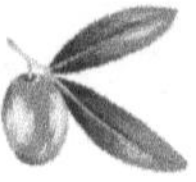

Chapter 8

Meal Planning and Prep

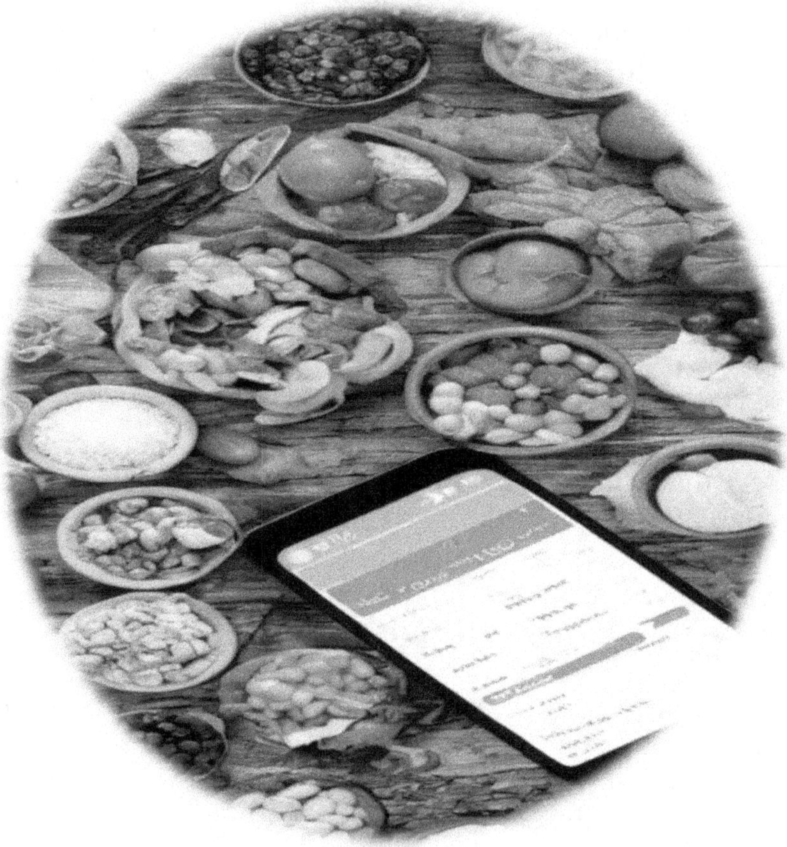

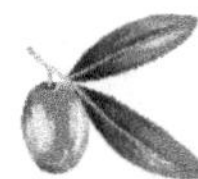

Meal planning and prepping can help you save time, money, and stress in the kitchen. Here are some tips and strategies for meal planning and prepping:

Plan your meals ahead of time: Take some time each week to plan out your meals for the week ahead. This can help you save time and money at the grocery store, and ensure that you have healthy and satisfying meals ready to go.

Batch cook: Batch cooking involves making large batches of food at once, then portioning them out for later use. This can be a great way to save time and ensure that you always have healthy meals on hand. Some great batch-cooking recipes include chili, soups, stews, and casseroles.

Use freezer-friendly recipes: Freezer-friendly recipes are meals that can be made ahead of time and frozen for later use. This can be a great way to save time and ensure that you always have healthy meals on hand. Some great freezer-friendly recipes include lasagna, meatballs, and baked goods like muffins and bread.

Make the most of leftovers: Leftovers can be a great way to save time and reduce food waste. Consider using leftovers in creative ways, such as turning them into a salad or sandwich, or using them as a base for a new recipe.

Reduce food waste: Food waste is a major problem in our society, but there are many ways to reduce it. Consider shopping with a list, buying only what you need, and using up ingredients before they go bad. You can also consider composting food scraps to reduce waste and create nutrient-rich soil for your garden.

By incorporating these meal planning and prepping strategies into your routine, you can save time, money, and

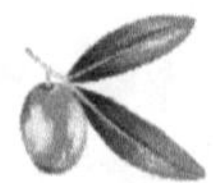

stress in the kitchen, while also ensuring that you have healthy and satisfying meals on hand.

Some good ways to use leftovers

Here are some good ways to use leftovers:

Turn them into a sandwich or wrap: Leftover meats or vegetables can be used as a filling for a sandwich or wrap. Add some fresh lettuce or other veggies and a spread like hummus or mustard for a tasty and satisfying meal.

Make a salad: Leftover vegetables, grains, or proteins can be used as a base for a salad. Add some fresh greens and a dressing for a healthy and nutritious meal.

Use them in a stir-fry: Leftover vegetables and meats can be used in a stir-fry with some fresh veggies and a sauce. Serve over rice or noodles for a quick and satisfying meal.

Make a soup or stew: Leftover meats, vegetables, and grains can be used as a base for a soup or stew. Add some broth and seasonings, and simmer until everything is heated through.

Make a frittata or quiche: Leftover vegetables and meats can be used as fillings for a frittata or quiche. Add some eggs, cheese, and herbs, and bake in the oven for a delicious and satisfying meal.

By using leftovers in creative ways, you can reduce food waste and save time and money in the kitchen. Plus, you'll have a variety of tasty and nutritious meals to enjoy throughout the week.

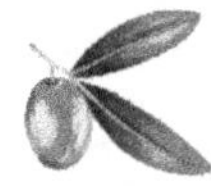

Other creative ways to use leftovers

Here are some other creative ways to use leftovers:

Make a pizza: Leftover meats and vegetables can be used as toppings for a homemade pizza. Add some sauce and cheese, and bake in the oven for a delicious and easy meal.

Use them in a quesadilla or burrito: Leftover meats and vegetables can be used as fillings for a quesadilla or burrito. Add some cheese and beans, and serve with salsa and sour cream for a tasty and filling meal.

Make a grain bowl: Leftover grains, meats, and vegetables can be used as a base for a grain bowl. Add some fresh greens, avocado, and a dressing for a healthy and satisfying meal.

Use them in a pasta dish: Leftover meats and vegetables can be added to a pasta dish for added flavor and nutrition. Add some sauce and cheese, and serve with a side salad for a complete meal.

Make a sandwich wrap: Leftover meats and vegetables can be used as a filling for a sandwich wrap. Add some cheese and a spread like hummus or mustard, and wrap it up for a portable and tasty meal.

By using leftovers in creative ways, you can save time and money in the kitchen while also reducing food waste. Plus, you'll have a variety of delicious and nutritious meals to enjoy throughout the week.

Make a pasta dish with leftover vegetables.

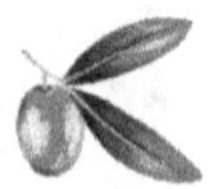

Making a pasta dish with leftover vegetables is a great way to use up your leftovers and create a quick and tasty meal. Here's a simple recipe to get you started:

Ingredients:

- 8 oz. pasta (any type you prefer)
- 2 cups of leftover vegetables (such as roasted bell peppers, zucchini, eggplant, or mushrooms)
- 2 cloves of garlic, minced
- 2 tablespoons of olive oil
- Salt and pepper to taste
- Parmesan cheese (optional)

Instructions:

01- Cook the pasta according to the package instructions until al dente. Drain and set aside.

02- In a large skillet, heat the olive oil over medium-high heat. Add the minced garlic and sauté for 1-2 minutes until fragrant.

03- Add the leftover vegetables to the skillet and cook for 3-4 minutes until heated through.

04- Add the cooked pasta to the skillet and toss to combine with the vegetables. Season with salt and pepper to taste.

05-If desired, top with grated Parmesan cheese before serving.

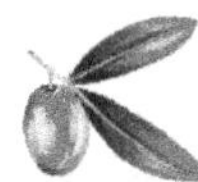

This pasta dish is a great way to use up leftover vegetables and create a quick and satisfying meal. You can customize it with your favorite vegetables and seasonings, and add a protein like chicken or shrimp if desired.

Other types of pasta dishes can I make with leftover vegetables:

There are many types of pasta dishes you can make using leftover vegetables. Here are a few ideas:

Pasta Primavera: This classic Italian dish combines pasta with fresh, seasonal vegetables like zucchini, bell peppers, and cherry tomatoes. The vegetables are sautéed in olive oil and garlic, then tossed with cooked pasta and Parmesan cheese.

Pesto Pasta: Pesto is a flavorful sauce made with fresh herbs like basil, garlic, and pine nuts. You can use leftover vegetables like roasted red peppers or cherry tomatoes to add extra flavor and texture to the dish. Toss the cooked pasta with the pesto and vegetables, then top with grated Parmesan cheese.

Vegetable Lasagna: Lasagna is a hearty and filling pasta dish that's perfect for using up leftover vegetables. Layer cooked lasagna noodles with a mixture of ricotta cheese, tomato sauce, and leftover vegetables like spinach, zucchini, and mushrooms. Top with mozzarella cheese and bake in the oven until bubbly and golden.

Spaghetti Carbonara: Carbonara is a creamy and indulgent pasta dish made with bacon, egg yolks, and Parmesan cheese. You can add leftover vegetables like roasted Brussels sprouts

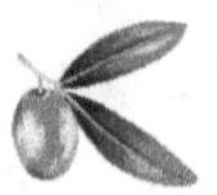

or sautéed mushrooms to the dish for extra flavor and nutrition.

Pasta Salad: Pasta salad is a refreshing and versatile dish that can be made with any leftover vegetables you have on hand. Cook the pasta according to the package instructions, then toss it with the vegetables, a simple vinaigrette, and some fresh herbs. Serve cold or at room temperature for a perfect summer meal.

These are just a few examples of the many types of pasta dishes you can make with leftover vegetables. Get creative and experiment with different combinations to find your favorite recipe!

*** Conclusion ***

The Mediterranean diet is more than just a way of eating, it's a lifestyle. This cookbook is a comprehensive guide to cooking delicious and healthy Mediterranean meals at home. With a focus on whole, nutrient-dense foods, this diet can help you feel your best and reduce your risk of chronic disease. Let this cookbook be your guide to a healthier and more flavorful way of eating.

While the Mediterranean diet is not a cure-all for chronic diseases, it has been shown to have many health benefits and may help prevent or manage certain conditions. Studies have found that following a Mediterranean-style diet can lower your risk of heart disease, stroke, type 2 diabetes, and certain types of cancer. The diet is rich in fruits,

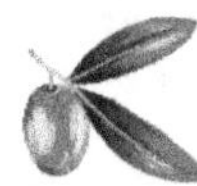

vegetables, whole grains, legumes, nuts, seeds, and healthy fats such as olive oil, and low in processed and unhealthy foods. This combination of nutrient-dense foods and healthy fats may help reduce inflammation, improve cholesterol levels, and support overall health and well-being. While it is important to consult with a healthcare professional for medical advice and specific treatment, following a Mediterranean-style diet can be a tasty and healthy way to support your health.

www.ingramcontent.com/pod-product-compliance
Lightning Source LLC
Chambersburg PA
CBHW050840260726

48660CB00006B/2354